Learning to care

on the

GYNAECOLOGY WARD

Wendy Simons
SRN, CERT ED

Clinical Nurse Specialist/Clinical Teacher,
Princess Anne Hospital, Southampton

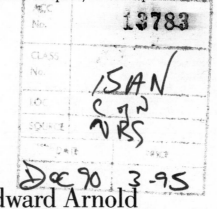
Edward Arnold
A division of Hodder & Stoughton
LONDON   MELBOURNE   AUCKLAND

LEARNING TO CARE SERIES

General Editors

JEAN HEATH, MED, BA, SRN, SCM, CERT ED
National Health Learning Resources Unit,
Sheffield

SUSAN E NORMAN, SRN, DN CERT, RNT
Senior Tutor, The Nightingale School,
West Lambeth Health Authority

© 1985 by W. Simons

First published in Great Britain 1985
Reprinted 1988

British Library Cataloguing in Publication Data

Simons, Wendy
    Learning to care on the gynaecology ward. –
    (Learning to care series)
    1. Gynecologic nursing
    I. Title   II. Series
    618.1'0024613   RG105

    ISBN 0 340 37000 9

Whilst the advice and information in this book is believed to be
true and accurate at the date of going to press, neither the author
nor the publisher can accept any legal responsibility or liability
for any errors or omissions that may be made.

Typeset in 10/11pt Trump Mediaeval by Rowland
Phototypesetting Limited, Bury St Edmunds, Suffolk. Printed
and bound in Great Britain for Edward Arnold, the educational,
academic and medical publishing division of Hodder and
Stoughton Limited, 41 Bedford Square, London WC1B 3DQ by
Richard Clay Limited, Bungay, Suffolk.

EDITORS' FOREWORD

In most professions there is a traditional gulf between theory and its practice, and nursing is no exception. The gulf is perpetuated when theory is taught in a theoretical setting and practice is taught by the practitioner.

This inherent gulf has to be bridged by students of nursing, and publication of this series is an attempt to aid such bridge building.

It aims to help relate theory and practice in a meaningful way whilst underlining the importance of the person being cared for.

It aims to introduce students of nursing to some of the more common problems found in each new area of experience in which they will be asked to work.

It aims to de-mystify some of the technical language they will hear, putting it in context, giving it meaning and enabling understanding.

PREFACE

This book is intended to help all nurses learning to care on the Gynaecology ward. It has given me great pleasure to write as I have long felt that there is a scarcity of books at the right level, treating patients as people with lives outside the hospital walls.

I hope that this book will help the nurses using it to relate the theory in the book to the practice seen on the wards. The questions and suggestions for further reading at the end of each chapter are there to enhance the learning experience in a way otherwise beyond the scope of this book.

I would like to thank Mr Jeremy Evans for his invaluable comments and suggestions.

The book is dedicated to all my students, past and present, for teaching me so much.

CONTENTS

Introduction

Nursing on the Gynaecology ward should be a happy and rewarding experience.

Gynaecology is defined as the study of the diseases of women, and therefore does not include childbirth, as this is a normal physiological function.

Most of the patients on the Gynaecology ward are between 16 and 60 years old, as many of the problems that arise are connected either with menstruation or fertility.

Patients are admitted to the hospital either as a routine or non-urgent admission, in which case they will have been seen by the gynaecologist in the Outpatients Department and put on the waiting list for admission, or they come in as an urgent admission sent by their general practitioner or by the Accident and Emergency Department. However they have arrived on the ward, patients will most likely be anxious or frightened, not only about their health, but about their families and perhaps their jobs, as well as by the alien environment of the hospital.

Women coming into hospital are often as worried about their homes and families as they are about the problem that has brought them there.

It should be clearly recognised that a disorder of the female reproductive system, whether it affects future fertility or not, whether it is a malignant growth or not, may also have a profound psychological effect on the patient. Many women consciously or unconsciously feel that their womanhood is being threatened and that their future role in life may be changed, and they react to this in many ways; some women cover their fears by talking too much, others by becoming withdrawn or dependent. Understanding some of the reasons for this will help you to give sympathetic nursing care.

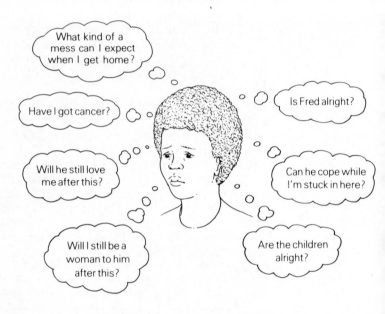

The continuing development of your interpersonal skills is very important in gynaecological nursing.

You will need to get to know your patients so that you can be sensitive to their needs, you will need knowledge and an understanding of the patient's condition, you will need the ability to sit and listen and you will need to have considered your own feelings and responses towards such topics as abortion and sexuality. Some patients may feel that their nurse is the only person in whom they can confide fears or worries of an intimate and personal nature, so it is important that you are able to listen without making judgments or betraying embarrassment.

One factor which may make getting to know your patient difficult is that most gynaecological patients are in hospital for quite a short time. Their length of stay can vary according to the patient's age and type of operation, from one day to as much as 12 weeks. The majority of patients, undergoing hysterectomy for example, will remain in hospital for 6 to 10 days. (See the glossary of terms at the end of this chapter.)

In order to give sympathetic skilled nursing care, a full nursing assessment must be made as soon as possible after admission.

The nursing assessment will take into account the psychological, social and spiritual needs of the patient as well as her physical needs. It is essential to find out how much the patient understands about her own body and present health problem, so that appropriate explanations can be made. The patient should be encouraged to talk and to ask questions; it is very helpful if this first interview is carried out in a private area, as there are many women who do not understand the terms we use or the consequences of the operation they are about to have, and are afraid to look foolish in front of others or waste your time by asking. It could be, also, that the subject under discussion is one which is particularly delicate or sensitive to the patient.

A very large proportion of women have suffered at some time of their lives with a gynaecological disorder, especially those disorders concerned with early pregnancy or menstruation. You will need to be alert to the fact that your patient may have been given a number of incorrect, misleading ideas or old wives' tales about her condition before she arrives on the ward.

On the Gynaecology ward you will be nursing many women who have had apparently the same operation for different reasons and it is important that you understand the reasons why each individual has had the operation as well as the operation itself if you are going to give good nursing care. Patients on the ward often compare their progress with the progress of the patient in the next bed, and become upset or worried because they are proceeding differently. Armed with this knowledge you will be able to explain that each person is an individual and responds differently to illness, and will therefore have a different rate of recovery. Women of many different ethnic groups may be patients in a British hospital and it is as well to recognise that they may all have differing ways of coping with a hysterectomy or with pain, and that they may have particular religious or cultural needs.

It may appear from this that gynaecology deals exclusively with surgery, but this is not so. Patients may have some very sophisticated investigations and treatment in the Outpatients Department, and they may be admitted to the ward for medical treatment such as antibiotic therapy for pelvic inflammatory disease or investigations and treatment of threatened abortion.

Gynaecology, although dealing with a fairly limited area of study has great variety and impinges on many other subjects.

While learning to care on the Gynaecology ward you will also be gaining some insight into these related topics.

How much of the nursing care you will give and how much you will observe only, depends on your own hospital and the stage of training you have reached by the time you are allocated to the Gynaecology ward.

Different wards have different learning objectives for their nurse learners. The

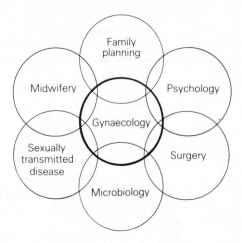

gynaecological one will probably include these:

1 *Assessment*

To carry out a nursing assessment of a newly admitted patient, both from the waiting list and as an urgent admission. There are several ways of doing this and it is probable that your hospital will have decided which one you should use; however the feature which most methods have in common is that they are a systematic process for establishing the patient's ability to carry out the activities of daily living, and using a system helps to ensure that nothing is forgotten.

The patient should be shown around the ward if she is mobile, including toilet areas, introduced to ward staff and other patients and informed of the daily routine. You should make sure that she knows where she can make a telephone call or buy a magazine; it is really the small homely details that will enable your patient to relax and feel at ease.

You will need to perform, record and report certain routine observations which will include:

Temperature
Pulse
Blood pressure
Urinalysis
Date of last menstrual period
Character of vaginal loss if present
Weight

Remember to explain to your patient why these observations are being made, otherwise it can be very alarming! Remember, too, that the patient's relatives may need some advice or assistance before they go home after accompanying the patient to the ward.

2 Planning care

In planning care you will need to be able to identify the patient's nursing needs or problems and to be able to set reasonable, measurable goals, discussing them as far as possible with the patient. Remember to set times or dates when the effectiveness of the care given can be evaluated.

3 Giving care

You will need to be able to care for your patient before, during and after special investigations and procedures. This means that you should be able to give an explanation to your patient in terms suited to her understanding and to give any preparatory or after care that is necessary. You may also be required to assist the doctor during some procedures, when your presence can be a great comfort to the patient. You will also be expected to observe your patient and report to the nurse in charge of the ward when this procedure is finished and your patient has been made comfortable.

You will need to know how to prepare patients for operation, which may involve giving simple explanations or asking a senior nurse or doctor to clarify certain points. The physical preparation for a gynaecological operation, although sometimes stressful to the patient, does not usually involve lengthy procedures such as a rectal washout. The gynaecologist is responsible for obtaining the patient's consent to the operation, and in the case of sterilisation it is considered desirable to obtain the consent of her husband as well.

You will need to be able to perform a vulval shave, give suppositories or an enema. Patients are very rarely given vaginal douches or vaginal packing prior to surgery.

You will need to be able to assess the patient's condition on return to the ward after an operation, and this will include:

Observations of vaginal loss

Observations of vaginal packs if used

The patient will be cared for by members of many different disciplines such as doctors, physiotherapists and nurses, but it is the nurse who is in continual contact with the patient longest. The nurse's role therefore is an important one, especially with regard to monitoring, reporting and communicating about the patient's well being to the other participants in her care.

During the postoperative phase you will be learning to incorporate the doctor's instructions into the planning and carrying out of detailed, personalised care which may include caring for the following:

An intravenous infusion

A urinary catheter (either urethral or suprapubic)

A wound drain (vacuum, corrugated, other)

Clips or other types of wound closure

A vaginal pack

Patients are usually in the Gynaecological ward such a short time that the ward nurses will be considering her return to the community very early in her hospital stay. Plans will be made which may include:

Teaching the patient and her relatives to prevent and recognise complications.

Giving very specific advice about the resumption of the activities of daily living, and checking that the information has been understood.

Encouraging the patient's questions.

Liaising with community nurses to provide further care.

Arranging a visit to a convalescent home.

4 Evaluating care

Evaluation is done during the patient's hospital stay to check that the care given is having the desired effect, so that changes can be made if the care is ineffective. However evaluation of care can also be performed after the patient has gone home so that the care in its entirety can be reviewed and plans made if necessary to try improvements on another occasion.

During your allocation to the Gynaecology ward observe the way in which the ward nurses care for a distressed patient or relative. Don't be afraid to put your arm around or hold the hand of someone who is upset. Take note of those actions which seem most helpful at the time and at an appropriate moment you may find it useful to discuss these with the nurse concerned. Remember that you don't have to know all the answers to be of comfort.

In summary gynaecological nursing is:
Providing Understanding; Support; Empathy; Expertise; Explanation
to patients with
Menstrual disorders; Pelvic infection; Disorders of early pregnancy; Fibromyoma; Uterovaginal prolapse; Infertility; Cancer; Endometriosis; Needing sterilisation
Who may need

Cervical smear	Dilatation and curettage
Vaginal examination	Laparoscopy
Ultrasound examination	Cone biopsy of cervix
High vaginal swab	Salpingectomy
Vulval hygiene	Oophorectomy
Removal of vaginal pack	Marsupialisation of
Removal of suture material	Bartholin's cyst
Care of wound drains	Hysterectomy
Urethral catheterisation	Vaginal repairs
Catheter care	Vulvectomy
Family help	Termination of pregnancy
Health education	Tubal surgery

Who may feel
Frightened of the hospital
Worried about a change of body image
Worried about their family
Stupid because they don't know what is happening
Relieved that a problem can be solved
Frightened of being infertile or having cancer

Glossary

Abortion	A condition where the products of conception are expelled from the uterus before the 28th week of pregnancy
Amenorrhoea	Absence of menstruation
Bartholin's glands	Small glands just inside the posterior aspect of the labia majora, which secrete a mucoid substance during sexual excitement

Cervical excitation	Pain occurring when the cervix is moved
Cervical os	The opening to the cervical canal
Cervix	The narrow portion of the uterus that forms its entrance and which protrudes into the vagina
Colporrhaphy	Vaginal repair
Colposcopy	Examination of the cervix by a low-powered binocular microscope
Cystocele	Prolapse of the bladder affecting the anterior vaginal wall
Dilatation and curettage	A diagnostic operation in which the cervix is dilated with instruments so that fragments of endometrium can be curetted and examined in the laboratory
Dysmenorrhoea	Painful menstrual periods
Dyspareunia	Difficult or painful coitus
Ectopic pregnancy	Pregnancy outside the uterine cavity
Enterocele	Prolapse of the gut affecting the posterior vaginal wall
Fibroids	Correctly called fibromyoma, these are benign growths arising from the muscle layer of the uterus
Fundus	That part of the uterus which lies above the insertion of the Fallopian tubes
Hydatidiform mole	An abnormal growth, usually benign, arising from placental (chorionic) tissue
Hysterectomy	Removal of the uterus
Laparoscopy	An operation where the contents of the pelvic cavity are viewed through a telescopic instrument called a laparoscope
Marsupialisation	The making of a false pocket usually describing the draining of an abcess of Bartholin's gland
Menarche	The onset of menstrual periods
Menopause	The cessation of menstrual periods
Myomectomy	Removal of fibroids

Oophorectomy	Removal of an ovary
Pessary	This may be either a device to keep the uterus in place or a vaginal medication rather like a suppository
Postmenopausal bleeding	Vaginal bleeding after the menopause
Procidentia	Complete prolapse of the uterus such that the fundus of the uterus is at the level of or beyond the introitus (entrance to vagina)
Prolapse	Displacement of one or more of the pelvic organs
Rectocele	Prolapse of the rectum affecting the posterior vaginal wall
Salpingectomy	Removal of the Fallopian tube
Shirodkar's suture	A purse string suture placed around the cervix in the case of an incompetent cervix
Termination of pregnancy	Abortion induced by surgical or medical means
Urethrocele	Prolapse of the urethra affecting the anterior vaginal wall
Ultrasound examination	An investigation in which a picture is built up from the differing times echoes take to bounce back from structures of varying density
Vulvectomy	Removal of the vulva

2 Christine Williams is admitted to the ward with a menstrual disorder

HISTORY

When Christine Williams started to have very heavy periods, it seemed as if not one thing in her life was going well.

Christine is 27 years old and works as a hairdresser in a salon in the town. She used to really enjoy going to work but lately has come to dread it. She and her fiancé John had been saving to get married until a few months ago when they had gone to a party given by one of Christine's colleagues. Not long after this John had broken off their engagement and started to go out with Christine's colleague. Unfortunately Christine and John had been sharing a flat which had been John's in the first instance so that Christine had to move out.

It was some months after this that Christine started to be troubled by menstrual periods which although occurring at regular intervals were very heavy and sometimes produced clots. This condition is called menorrhagia.

There are many types of menstrual disorders, and it should be remembered that they may have different causes. Three frequently mentioned types are:
Menorrhagia (as above)

Amenorrhoea – absence of menstrual periods, which may be further classified into primary amenorrhoea (when a woman has never had a period) and secondary (when a woman has had menstrual periods but they have now ceased)

Dysmenorrhoea – difficult or painful periods, which may be further classified into primary dysmenorrhoea (where the woman has always had the problem) and secondary (where the woman has initially experienced painless periods but has now developed dysmenorrhoea)

History taking will include:
The age of the patient at the menarche

The amount, duration and frequency of menstrual periods

Discussion of the patient's background and environment, contraceptive history if relevant, marital or emotional problems

A summary of her obstetric and any other medical history especially any tendency to blood disorders.

Christine's menorrhagia was sufficiently bad to make it difficult for her to remain walking about all day at the salon during a period, and in the interval between periods she began to feel very weak and listless. Eventually after discussing it with her mother, Christine went to see her G.P., who suggested that she should have an appointment to see a gynaecologist at the local hospital.

When Christine attends the Outpatient Department for her first visit she is very nervous but relieved that something will be done to help her.

The gynaecologist takes a careful, sympathetic history.

The gynaecologist performs a physical examination, which will include the patient's entire body not just the genital tract. The calm presence of the nurse during the examination should reassure Christine during what may be an embarrassing experience and may help her to feel more relaxed and less anxious.

During physical examination in the Gynaecology Clinic, the special points to be aware of are the development of secondary sexual characteristics, and the normal distribution of hair, which are dependent on an adult female's production of hormones

The gynaecologist will perform a vaginal examination which usually includes both a bimanual examination (see next chapter) and a speculum examination. This is performed to estimate the size of the uterus and to detect whether or not the uterus is in the correct position of anteversion, that is, lying tilted towards the bladder and symphysis pubis, and whether or not the uterus is mobile, which it should be. The presence of any adnexal masses may also be detected.

The speculum examination should enable the gynaecologist to tell whether or not the patient has a lesion such as a cervical polyp or erosion. Often the gynaecologist may wish to take a cervical smear to detect any abnormal cells on the cervix.

Speculum examination

There are many types of vaginal speculum, but there are two which are perhaps used more often than others and these are called respectively Sim's speculum (used primarily to assess prolapse) and Cuscoe's speculum (used primarily to inspect the cervix). A good light is needed to use either effectively, and some come with a built-in light source, but the majority do not.

Blood tests:
A haemoglobin test will show whether Christine has become anaemic. Sometimes the gynaecologist will request that blood is taken for a full blood count to see to what extent the intermittent haemorrhage has produced changes in the blood cells. He may ask for coagulation studies or possibly thyroid function tests as abnormal thyroid function can cause menorrhagia. There are also hormone assays, but these will probably be done only if it is apparent at the time of the examination that there is a hormone imbalance or if the patient's complaint is one of infertility.

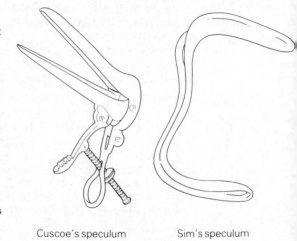

Cuscoe's speculum   Sim's speculum

Christine also has a sample of her blood taken for testing.

The Gynaecologist tells Christine that the best diagnostic procedure for her condition is dilatation and curettage, which although a minor procedure is performed in the operating theatre with the patient anaesthetised. It is explained to Christine that the maximum amount of information will be gained from this procedure if it is performed during the second half of her menstrual cycle when the endometrium can be examined to determine its response to the hormones in circulation at that time. In the meantime she is asked to keep a careful record of her menstrual periods, their frequency, duration and the character of the blood loss. It is not always easy for the gynaecologist to assess menstrual loss as people's perceptions of what is or is not a heavy loss vary considerably. Christine is asked to count the number of sanitary towels she uses and to note whether they are stained or soaked through.

When Christine receives her appointment to come to the hospital she is asked to come the day before her operation. This will enable the anaesthetist and gynaecologist to see her to check her fitness for the operation and also to allow Christine to settle into the ward and to meet some of the nursing staff.

ADMISSION TO THE WARD

Christine arrives for admission one Monday afternoon, and notices to her surprise that there seem to be a lot of other patients for admission that day. She tells the ward receptionist of her arrival. Then a nurse, introducing herself as Liz Parker, shows Christine to a bed. Liz asks Christine to change into her night dress and to unpack her belongings into the bedside locker. When this is done, Christine is shown around the ward and has the ward routine described to her. Liz has to take some routine observations and she explains the reasons for these so that Christine won't become alarmed. Observations of temperature, pulse and blood pressure are taken even though Christine is not ill, to establish her own normal readings before she is subjected to an anaesthetic or an operation. She is asked

Understanding the normal menstrual cycle will help you to understand some of the factors involved in menstrual disorders.

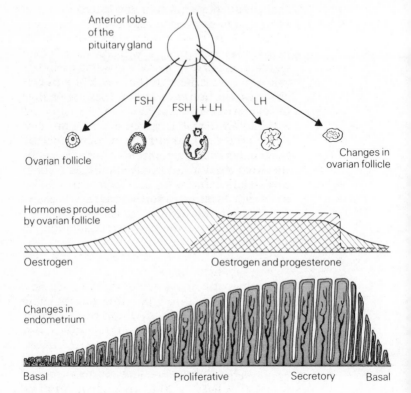

FSH - Follicular stimulating hormone
LH - Luteinising hormone

about the first day of her last menstrual period and about any vaginal discharge, should any be present, as this information can be helpful when the curettings from the endometrium are examined under the microscope.

Liz and Christine discuss Christine's needs while she is in the hospital so that a full nursing assessment can be made and her care planned. Liz is able to answer some of Christine's questions, such as the length of time she will be in the hospital, and the likely time that the operation will take place, and also that the gynaecologist and anaesthetist will see her later in the day. Christine is introduced to the other patients in her room, who have also been admitted today and they are all offered a cup of tea. Liz asks all of them to call a nurse if they wish to pass urine, as a specimen of urine is needed for a test for abnormalities. This may include a test for protein, which could indicate a urinary tract infection, or a test for sugar, which might indicate that the patient has diabetes mellitus.

All the patients are encouraged to ask any questions, and those that the nursing staff cannot answer are passed on to the gynaecologist. Gynaecology is a subject which has attracted a large number of articles in the popular press and television programmes, most of which are excellent, but sometimes the patient has not fully understood them or has wrongly assumed that the article or programme refers to her own case.

NURSING CARE

Initial stages

Christine was right that there were a lot of patients being admitted that day, because they are all patients who are being admitted from the waiting list rather than urgently. Christine is one of eight who are scheduled for operation the following day, and she feels comforted by the company of her fellow patients, and starts to strike up a friendship with a girl of about her own age in the next bed.

Later that day Christine meets the doctors and is examined and pronounced fit for the operation. Liz returns and is able to alleviate one of her fears at once by explaining that patients having a dilatation and curettage do not need to be shaved. She also explains that Christine must have nothing to eat after midnight as the operation will take place at 9 o'clock, and then describes the operation procedure.

That night Christine's mother and a friend visit bringing fruit and magazines. Christine feels rather a fraud as she does not feel ill, but her new friend in the next bed, who has been a patient before, laughs and tells her to make the most of it. Christine is reassured as much by the conversation of the other patients on the ward as by the assurances of the nurses and the doctors, and eventually sleeps well.

The next morning Christine wakes and has a shower as part of the preparation for theatre. She is then given a white gown before returning to her bed. Two nurses bring her pre-medication of Metoclopramide 10mg and Diazepam 10mg to be taken orally, but as they explain to her, there are certain checks that are made to ensure her safety during the operation and these are carried out before the drugs are given. Both nurses observe that her identity bands are correct, that her consent form has been signed, that she has no jewellery or underwear on, and that she has no dentures to be removed. They mention that this is all routine pre-operative procedure. Both nurses stay with Christine while she takes the tablets and ask her to call a nurse if there is anything at all that she needs.

Christine now has about an hour to wait

The start of **dilatation and curettage** is a careful pelvic examination as a more thorough examination can be conducted while the patient is fully relaxed under the anaesthetic. The cervix is then dilated using graduated dilators until the internal os is sufficiently open to allow the passage of a uterine sound and a curette. The former is used to check the size of the uterine cavity. The latter is used to remove pieces of endometrium which are sent to the laboratory for examination, and can also detect irregularities of the uterine cavity.

before she goes to the operating theatre for a dilatation and curettage.

NURSING CARE

Rehabilitation

After the operation is finished Christine is taken to the recovery area where she stays, under observation, until the anaesthetist is satisfied that she is fit enough to be returned to the ward.

Liz comes to collect her, and although she is very sleepy Christine is grateful for seeing a familiar face. Once they are back in the ward and Christine has been made comfortable, Liz takes a series of observations like the ones noted on admission to ensure that Christine is continuing to recover from the anaesthetic and the operation.

Pulse

Blood pressure

Vaginal loss – a certain amount of vaginal bleeding is expected after a curettage operation.

Christine's observations are all within normal limits. As she is now resting peacefully, it is not considered necessary to disturb her by carrying out further observations. Liz makes sure that the nurse call system is within easy reach of Christine's hand before she goes to attend to other patients.

Christine sleeps well until tea time and wakes up hungry. She is helped to have a wash, brush her hair, clean her teeth, and to put on her own clothes again, and after this is done she has a cup of tea and a biscuit. Liz accompanies Christine to the lavatory when she is ready to pass urine so that should she feel weak there is help at hand. Liz is also able to reassure Christine that if some extra blood loss appears at this time it will probably be blood which has pooled in the vagina while she was lying down rather than fresh bleeding.

Christine feels rather tired when she gets out of bed and is very relieved to get back into it again. This is the main reason why it was suggested to her that she stay overnight after the operation, as many women feel the need to rest after an anaesthetic.

Planning discharge

By morning however Christine feels ready to go home. As her observations have been within normal limits both morning and evening the only nursing care which she still needs is the advice prior to discharge. The gynaecologist comes to see her before she goes home in order to discuss the operation findings with her and to make a final check on her fitness to go home.

Christine is allowed to go home with an appointment to attend the clinic in six weeks' time.

A nurse takes time to discuss with Christine some points which may arise after she has left the hospital.

Advice on discharge:
To return to her work when she feels ready and that this may take up to a week after the operation.
To use sanitary towels for her next period rather than tampons as the cervix has been opened and it is wise to reduce the chance of introducing infection to a minimum.
Her next period may be either early or late and the amount of loss will be variable.
This operation may effect a temporary cure.

Care following discharge

When Christine returns to the Outpatient Department in six weeks' time, the gynaecologist will have the report on the curettings. If there is no organic cause for her menorrhagia, then the conclusion will be that her emotional state is acting on the pituitary gland. In young women menorrhagia usually resolves spontaneously. In order to make life more tolerable Christine may be offered hormone preparations to bring her cycle back to normal or non-hormone preparations such as Danazol or Epsikapron which, although acting in different ways, will have much the same effect. If she is anaemic she may be offered iron tablets although once her menstrual loss has diminished she may regain a normal haemoglobin level naturally.

Christine may be worried by the findings or by the advice given and time should be spent by the doctor and nurse together to be sure that Christine fully understands the likely course of events and effects of any treatment offered.

| TEST YOURSELF |

Check with your Tutor or Ward Sister that you understand the questions and have answered them fully.

1 Discuss the part played by emotional factors in menstrual disorders.

2 Is there an element of risk in the free interchange of ideas between fellow patients? If so, what should you do about it?

3 What is the value of admitting patients to the hospital the day before surgery?

4 Find out and take note of the pre- and postoperative care given to patients in your own hospital.

5 What action should Liz take if she finds that Christine's postoperative observations are not within normal limits, for example, that her blood pressure has become very low and her pulse very fast?

FURTHER READING

ABBRO, F. 1984. Periods of Misery. *Nursing Mirror*, **159** (2).

DALTON, K. 1983. *Once a month*. London: Fontana.

GOUGH, H. 1982. Moody Blues. *Nursing Mirror*, March 17th.

RUTTER, M. 1984. Intermenstrual Bleeding. *Nursing Times*, Feb. 29th.

3 Linda Jones has a threatened abortion

Linda Jones is 20 years old and is married to David. They rent the top floor flat of a large Victorian house a little way from the shops, with friends and family living nearby. Both are working, David as a salesman and Linda as a shop assistant.

They were not planning to start a family until they had saved some money and moved to a small house with a garden, but when Linda suspected that she might be pregnant, they were both delighted. Linda and David had the pregnancy confirmed by their G.P. and started to make plans for the baby's arrival.

Six weeks later, when Linda is 12 weeks pregnant, she starts to have a mild backache while working in the shop. On inspection she finds that she has lost a small amount of bright red blood, apparently from her vagina. She is

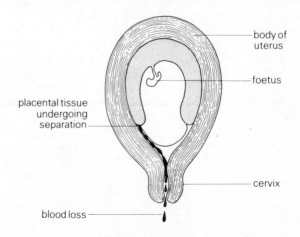

body of uterus

foetus

placental tissue undergoing separation

cervix

blood loss

very frightened and leaves work straight away, and telephones her Doctor who arranges for admission to the local hospital. He diagnoses her condition as a threatened abortion.

Abortion is defined as the expulsion from the uterus of the products of conception before the 28th week of pregnancy. This date is an important one to remember as after this a foetus is said to be viable; that is, capable of independent life.

Types of Spontaneous Abortion

Threatened Abortion
may become
either ————————→ *Complete Abortion*
or
Incomplete Abortion
If this happens three or
more consecutive times it is
called *Habitual Abortion*

Inevitable Abortion

Normal Pregnancy

If the foetus dies inside the uterus and is not expelled it is called a *Missed Abortion*

ADMISSION TO THE WARD

Linda is very distressed when she arrives on the ward; as well as her fear of losing the baby, she has not been able to contact her husband and it is the first time that she has ever been in a hospital. A nurse greets Linda on her arrival, introducing herself as Liz Parker, and undertakes to telephone David as soon as Linda is settled into bed and the doctor has been informed of her arrival. Liz helps Linda into her nightdress and into bed, explaining the nurse call system as she does so. Liz has certain essential observations to make and she explains the reasons for these as she does them.

Observations of pulse, blood pressure and vaginal loss are made so that the safety of Linda's pregnancy or otherwise can be ascertained. Although it may upset Linda to know that the more blood she loses the less likely the pregnancy is to survive, it is still more worrying for her to have no idea what is hap-

Bimanual examination: the patient lies in the Dorsal position, that is, lying on her back with her head supported by one pillow, and with her knees flexed and apart.
The doctor uses one hand to

examine the vagina and cervix while gently pushing the fundus of the uterus downward with the other, so that the cervix comes within reach of the examining fingers and can be easily felt.

Signs and symptoms of a threatened abortion: uterine bleeding, usually bright red initially, changing to dark brown. There may or may not be slight lower abdominal pain or backache. Vaginal examination reveals that the cervical os is not dilated.

pening. Liz explains that her temperature is taken so that her own normal temperature will be known in case she should develop an infection with pyrexia. Observations which are made in order to establish the patient's own normal are called baseline observations. Linda's pulse will be raised above normal because of the bleeding and her anxiety.

Liz stays with Linda while the doctor talks to her and performs a bimanual examination. Linda's cervix is not open and the diagnosis of threatened abortion is confirmed.

The Doctor is able to tell Linda that there is a chance that the baby will be all right, and prescribes her treatment.

Once the medical treatment has been prescribed and it is apparent that Linda is comforted by the news, Liz and Sister devise a nursing care plan which identifies Linda's needs and states the best way of meeting them.

Meanwhile David has arrived and Liz leaves them alone together, after having made them a cup of tea.

NURSING CARE

Initial stages

Linda is nursed in bed until her vaginal bleeding stops. She is in no danger of developing pressure sores as she is able to move about in bed quite freely and also because she is young and fit. However Liz is aware that being confined to bed means that Linda must have everything she needs to hand and is careful to see that Linda has her books and knitting on her locker and that the nurse call system is within reach. She tells Linda that observations will be taken at four-hourly intervals and that she will pop in and out, but that any time

Medical treatment:
Blood tests for haemoglobin, group and Rhesus factor. The laboratory will also be asked to save the serum so that if Linda starts to bleed heavily it will take only a short time to commence a blood transfusion.

Urine is sent to the laboratory for a pregnancy test, although unfortunately this test is not very helpful as it will continue to be positive for some time after foetal death has occurred.

Linda would like something or is worried, she should call for a nurse.

Liz also warns Linda that she may find extra blood when passing urine but that she need not be alarmed as this is probably blood which has pooled in the vagina while she was lying down rather than fresh blood. Liz is careful to offer Linda a bowl to wash her face and hands at frequent intervals as well as when she uses the bed pan, because lying in bed makes people very hot and sticky.

At first Linda did not feel like eating anything, but Liz encouraged her to choose small, high fibre meals from the hospital menu. David often brought her some small delicacy from home to tempt her appetite as well. The high fibre diet is important for pregnant women are very liable to become constipated, as the movement of the gastrointestinal tract slows down during pregnancy. In Linda's case bedrest is an additional problem, as exercise would normally also contribute to a regular bowel motion. Liz explains to Linda that she must not strain at stool as this may stimulate

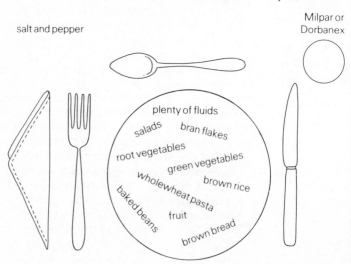

salt and pepper

Milpar or Dorbanex

plenty of fluids
salads   bran flakes
root vegetables
green vegetables
wholewheat pasta   brown rice
baked beans   fruit
brown bread

the uterus to contract so Linda is given a very mild aperient to eliminate any possibility of constipation.

During the first few hours after her admission Linda is in need of reassurance frequently, but as time goes on and her ultrasound examination confirms that all is well with the baby she becomes more relaxed.

Linda responds well to bed rest and after 48 hours the vaginal loss visible on her sanitary towel is much diminished and is pale brown which indicates that the loss is not fresh.

NURSING CARE

Rehabilitation

Linda is now allowed to get up to go to the bathroom and the lavatory, but remains on bed rest otherwise. Liz notices that Linda is becoming rather restless and makes an opportunity to sit and chat with her to try to find out the cause. It is soon revealed that Linda is now getting bored and feels that she could rest equally well at home. Liz tells Sister of this conversation and they discuss with the doctor the possibility of Linda being allowed home. Later that day when David visits, he and Linda talk with the doctor and they agree that Linda should not be at home resting alone. David says that he can have a week's holiday and then Linda's mother who lives close by will probably be able to be with her for most of the day. Linda will gradually reduce the amount of time she spends resting as she continues to improve. As the pregnancy continues and grows, Linda will be advised to rest in the afternoons anyway.

Planning discharge

Linda is given a lot of advice before she leaves the hospital.

Incomplete abortion:

A pregnant woman experiences vaginal bleeding which may be heavy and may contain clots

There may be cramping lower abdominal pain and backache

Blood is taken for Hb. blood group and save serum, and Rhesus factor

The patient is prepared for theatre and an *evacuation of retained products of conception* is performed

Before being allowed home the patient must have no signs or symptoms of an infection, a satisfactory Hb. level, have received family planning advice and have her Rhesus factor established. She is advised not to try to become pregnant again until she has had at least one normal period and feels psychologically ready to do so

Advice on discharge:

She may only do light work

She should rest for two hours every afternoon

She should eat a well balanced diet (it is a myth that pregnant women need to eat for two)

She should wear low heeled shoes and loose comfortable clothing

She should not smoke

She should wear a support brassiere

She and David should refrain from sexual intercourse until she has been told by the doctor that they may resume

She should not carry heavy items such as groceries

She may telephone the hospital at any time if she is worried

Linda goes home on the fifth day after her admission, with an appointment for the Outpatients Department in two weeks' time. A letter is sent to her G.P. immediately on her discharge informing him of her treatment.

Linda is one of the lucky ones. If you turn to the flow chart which tells you the possible outcomes of a threatened abortion, you can see that the alternative to a normal pregnancy is either a complete or an incomplete abortion. Approximately one in five pregnancies end in a spontaneous abortion, so it will be useful to you to have a brief summary of what might have happened to Linda.

A complete abortion means that the uterus is completely empty of all the products of conception and as such needs no treatment. In practice however it is difficult to know whether this has happened or if the uterus still contains some tissue. The latter case is called an incomplete abortion and the remaining tissue must be removed surgically as otherwise the uterus cannot stop bleeding and the uterine contents could become infected.

The Importance of the Rhesus Factor:
The Rhesus factor is always checked because a Rhesus negative mother who has a Rhesus positive partner may have conceived a Rhesus positive foetus. When the placental tissue separates from the uterine wall it is possible for the foetal and maternal blood to mix, and should this happen the mother's blood will start to form antibodies to the Rhesus positive blood. To stop this happening the mother will be prescribed and given an intramuscular dose of Rhesus immunoglobulins within 72 hours of the placental separation.

Some causes of early abortion (first 3 months):
Foetal abnormality
Pyrexia
Drugs or poisons
Hormone insufficiency
Uterine abnormality

This patient will not be in hospital very long and thus it is not easy for the nurse to tell that the patient may be going through some very deep and complex emotional changes. Many women feel bereaved or guilty by the spontaneous abortion. Sometimes an agency outside the immediate family circle may be able to help the couple to come to terms with their feelings. There are several self-help groups in this country and addresses where they can be contacted should be made available to the couple.

In many cases of spontaneous abortion no cause is found, but many women who have experienced a spontaneous abortion proceed to have a normal pregnancy soon afterwards.

TEST YOURSELF

Check with your Tutor or Ward Sister that you understand the questions and have answered them fully.

1 Describe the different types of abortion to a junior nurse.

2 Discuss the nurse's role in being with the doctor while a vaginal examination is carried out.

3 What types of behaviour may alert you to the fact that the patient is not able to cope with her current problems?

4 How can a nurse prevent a patient like Linda who is young and fit becoming bored with bed rest?

5 How would you discuss the further treatment that is advised after discharge from hospital, with Linda, or with David and

Linda together, and how would you set about it?

FURTHER READING

FRIEDMAN & GRADSTEIN. 1982. *Surviving Pregnancy Loss*. Boston: Little, Brown and Company.

OAKLEY, A., MCPHERSON, A. & ROBERTS, H. 1983. *Miscarriage*. London: Fontana.

RUTLEDGE, D. 1984. Inevitable Abortion. *Nursing Mirror*, **158** (6).

STEWART, A. 1984. Intrauterine Death. *Nursing Mirror*, **158** (6).

4 Debbie Smith has a termination of pregnancy

HISTORY

Debbie and Steve Smith's problem was not that Debbie was pregnant, they were quietly happy about that. No, the problem was that Debbie at about the 12th week of her pregnancy had contracted rubella (German measles). Debbie and Steve are aware that rubella caught in the first three months of pregnancy can cause foetal abnormality, but they are not sure what the chances are that their baby may be affected and if so what sort of abnormality might result.

Rubella in early pregnancy is one of the conditions which in law justifies termination of pregnancy. Debbie remembered that when she was at school there was a campaign to ensure that all school girls were immunised against rubella. She and her Mother were confident however that she had already had the illness, and in the event, Debbie had been away from school with influenza during the time that the immunisations had been given.

Debbie and Steve are a young couple living in a two bedroomed terrace house on a new housing estate. Steve has just been promoted to the post of charge nurse on a Psychogeriatric ward. Debbie is not working at the moment although she has worked as a typist. This pregnancy was planned as they both feel that they would like to have their family young.

Debbie's G.P. diagnoses her spotty rash as rubella and warns her of some of the possible

Rubella or German measles in the adult is often unrecognised as it is a mild illness, and the outward sign is a rash that may be thought to be an allergy and does not last long.

Chances of foetal abnormality occurring are: during the first 4 weeks of life (50%) during the next 4 weeks of life (20%) during the third 4 weeks of life (15%) Abnormalities that may result from infection can involve the brain, ears, eyes and heart.

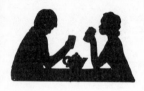

consequences to the baby. This comes as a shock to Debbie, and she is very tearful when she tells Steve that evening. They discuss it all evening and most of the night, and by morning they are reluctantly sure that if the baby was grossly abnormal they could not bear it. They are also thinking of the future as they hope to have more than one child, and if they had an abnormal baby they would not be able to cope with other children as well.

Debbie's G.P. has told her that unfortunately there are no tests that would reliably distinguish all abnormalities in the foetus. He is able to make an appointment to visit them before Steve goes to work on a late duty the following day. Debbie cannot come to the surgery in case she gives rubella to other patients.

Debbie, Steve and their G.P. have a long talk together about their feelings. The G.P. discusses with them the hazards of a termination of pregnancy, and also the way that they may feel after the termination has been performed, perhaps guilty, perhaps relieved, perhaps grieved as if this was a baby they had known a long time. Steve and Debbie are quite sure of their feelings, so their G.P. contacts the hospital for an early meeting with the gynaecologist, and arranges an appointment for the following week.

Debbie and Steve have a miserable weekend waiting for their appointment day, but they love each other and are able to be mutually supportive. When at last the day comes they go to the clinic together. The gynaecologist is prepared to spend a lot of time with them, to be absolutely sure that the decision they have reached is the right one for them. He finds that all aspects have been comprehensively discussed with them and that very little counselling is necessary.

Abortion is not undertaken lightly and there are many studies about pre- and post-abortion counselling.

Suction termination of pregnancy may be undertaken when the uterus is 12 weeks or less in size. The patient is taken to the operating theatre and her cervix is dilated with metal dilators. The contents of the uterus are then aspirated and sometimes the uterus is curetted in the conventional manner as well. The patient is allowed home as soon as she is well enough, has received family planning advice and has had her Rhesus factor checked.

The Abortion Act of 1967 allows termination of pregnancy to be carried out under the following provisions:

1 The continuance of the pregnancy would involve risk to the life of the pregnant woman greater than if the pregnancy were terminated.
2 The continuance of the pregnancy would involve risk of injury to the physical or mental health of the pregnant woman greater than if the pregnancy were terminated.
3 The continuance of the pregnancy would involve risk of injury to the physical or mental health of the existing children greater than if the pregnancy were terminated.
4 There is a substantial risk that if the child were born it would suffer from such physical or mental abnormalities as to be seriously handicapped.
5 To save the life of the pregnant woman.
6 To prevent grave permanent injury to the physical or mental health of the pregnant woman.

After the gynaecologist has taken a full history from Debbie, and a physical examination, he finds that her uterus is slightly too big for a suction termination of pregnancy.

The gynaecologist explains to Debbie that it would be dangerous for her to undergo this relatively simple procedure and that the abortion will be induced medically with prostaglandins, which will take anywhere between 12 and 24 hours, and that she may need a small operation afterwards to ensure that her uterus is empty.

Debbie is given an inpatient appointment for the following week, and she and Steve go home to wait for the time to come. It is sometimes possible for patients to be admitted straight from the Outpatient Department but only when the patient's need is very urgent, which is not so in Debbie's case.

ADMISSION
TO THE
WARD

Debbie is asked to come to the ward early in the morning. When she arrives she is admitted to a single room, and asked to undress and put her belongings into the bedside locker. Debbie discusses her needs while in hospital with Liz Parker so that a plan of care can be formulated. The nursing assessment is a far-reaching one, including such points as the fact that Debbie has recently had a rash, and it reveals Debbie's extreme nervousness. During the time that Liz spends with Debbie she takes her baseline observations, explaining them as she goes, asks for a specimen of urine to test, and is able to answer some of Debbie's questions.

Liz stays with Debbie while the doctor chats with her and asks Debbie to sign a consent form.

NURSING CARE

Initial stages

Once the procedure has started, and Debbie has been made comfortable, Liz will start a series of half-hourly observations, which will include: pulse, blood pressure, vaginal loss, presence of abdominal pain or contractions.

Debbie will only be allowed fluids during the procedure for safety reasons, so that if she starts to bleed heavily and needs to be taken to the operating theatre as an emergency, her stomach will be easy to empty. Debbie has brought some books with her but she finds that she cannot concentrate. She wishes Steve could remain with her, but although the hospital would allow him to stay, he has had to go to work. The ward nurses spend as much time as they can with her. Eventually, when Debbie starts having the lower abdominal pain and blood loss which indicate that the uterus is contracting, she is given a strong analgesia which also makes her sleepy.

Steve comes in when he has finished work and sits with her. At seven o'clock some pro-

ways, in the vagina, orally, intravenously, intra- or extra-amniotically.

Termination of pregnancy using extra-amniotic prostaglandins: Practical details of this procedure vary from gynaecologist to gynaecologist and therefore this is only a guide to the method used. The gynaecologist inserts a Foley catheter through the cervix into the space between the amniotic sac and the uterine wall, he attaches some tubing to this, which connects to a clockwork pump at the other end so that a controlled flow of prostaglandins is washing around the cervix and uterine wall all the time. An intravenous infusion may be set up containing oxytocin (Syntocinon).

The Conscience Clause: Any nurse who has a particular objection to caring for a patient having a therapeutic termination of pregnancy is permitted to

ducts of conception are passed. Debbie recognises that something has happened and rings for a nurse, who asks Steve to leave while she looks. As happens very frequently with abortion at this stage of gestation, the foetus is expelled but it is difficult to know whether or not there are products of conception left in the uterus. Liz calls the Sister and together they assure Debbie and Steve that the worst part is over, but that they think that when the doctor comes he will say that an evacuation of retained products is needed.

Debbie is seen by the doctor, and prepared for theatre. Later that evening she has an evacuation of retained products of conception under general anaesthetic. She is observed during the night for signs of fever or haemorrhage. By morning she is assessed as being well but hungry. Debbie's blood tests reveal that she has a Rhesus negative blood type, so she is prescribed and given Rhesus immunoglobulins before she leaves the hospital.

NURSING CARE

Planning Discharge

The Doctor sees Debbie and Steve before they leave the hospital to explain that they should wait before trying to conceive again at least until Debbie has had one normal period and feels emotionally ready. He advises them about family planning and resuming intercourse and also tells Debbie that she does not need a follow up appointment in the Outpatient Department unless she is worried after she is discharged.

Debbie is given some advice before she goes home.

exercise her right to refuse. Nurses employed to work on gynaecological wards should have had this question discussed well before they come to the ward as should learner nurses prior to an allocation to the Gynaecology ward.

However it is important to realise that no nurse can in law refuse to give care in an emergency to a patient having a termination of pregnancy.

Advice on discharge:

To use sanitary towels for her next menstrual period rather than tampons

Her next period may be either early or late

The present vaginal loss should diminish and turn brown within a few days, turning pinkish before stopping altogether

Should her vaginal discharge become heavy, bright red or offensive she should seek medical advice as this could indicate infection or retained products of conception

She should avoid intercourse for about four weeks to minimise any chance of an infection occurring while the cervix is open

To allow themselves to grieve as it is natural and healthy that they should

TEST YOURSELF

Check with your Tutor or Ward Sister that you understand the questions and have answered them fully.

1 Give examples of the conditions or circumstances to which the clauses of the Abortion Act might apply.

2 There are sometimes very controversial cases cited in the press, for example when a 16 year old girl has a termination of pregnancy performed without her parents' knowledge. Discuss the possible reasons why this situation may occur, and the nurse's role in preserving confidentiality.

3 Patients react in different ways to termination of pregnancy. Outline some of the range of emotional reactions that may occur.

4 Much has been said about counselling after abortion, particularly that patients do not come forward for counselling. Why do you think this may be?

FURTHER READING

BICHARD, G. & POWELL, S. 1982. Sense and Sensitivity. *Nursing Mirror*, April 14th.

BROOME, A. 1984. Abortion Counselling. *Nursing Mirror*, **158** (20).

GARDNER, R. S. G. 1975. *Abortion – the personal dilemma*. Exeter: The Paternoster Press.

HULME, H. 1983. Therapeutic Abortion and Nursing Care. *Nursing Times*, Oct. 12th.

5

Pauline King is admitted with acute pelvic inflammatory disease

HISTORY

Differential diagnoses may include:
Appendicitis
Pyelonephritis
Torsion of ovarian cyst
Ectopic pregnancy (this is an acute gynaecological emergency – see next chapter)
Pelvic inflammatory disease

Equipment prepared for an emergency admission:
The bed should have a drawer mackintosh and sheet (this is a gynaecological patient who may be bleeding vaginally)
A stethoscope and sphygmomano-meter

Pauline King was admitted to the Ward at 2 a.m. She had been feeling unwell and had experienced lower abdominal pain for several days, but on this day the pain had become gradually worse until by 11 p.m. she was in severe pain and very frightened. John, her husband, persuaded her that they should telephone their G.P. and he came to see her at half past midnight. He took Pauline's temperature, which was raised, and discussed her symptoms with her, and then told her that he thought she ought to go to the hospital to be observed and investigated.

Pauline was upset, but as the pain was still severe and she was very worried, she agreed to go. John quickly gathered together some of the things that she might need in hospital, while the G.P. organised an ambulance and talked to the doctor on duty at the hospital.

Pauline and John are in their early thirties, and they have a small interior decorating business, which they run themselves with some help. They have put off having children for the moment, so that they can make their business a going concern. Pauline has had a nagging lower abdominal pain for about a week, but dismissed it from her mind, thinking that it was probably her menstrual period that was due.

In the darkened quiet ward, the night nurse

A thermometer
Oxygen
A vomit bowl (a
patient with severe
abdominal pain
may feel sick
whatever the
cause)
Items for
performing a
vaginal
examination and
taking a swab for
culture
Items for setting up
an intravenous
infusion, including
syringes, needles
and specimen
containers for
sending blood
samples
All documents
needed such as
nursing assessment
form and care plan,
temperature chart
and fluid chart

Observations:
Pulse
Temperature
Blood pressure
The presence and
character of any
vaginal loss
The nature and
duration of pain

**Signs and
symptoms of pelvic
inflammatory
disease (acute):**
The pulse rate is
increased
The blood pressure
is slightly low
probably due to
pain
The temperature is
raised

receives the message that a patient is coming in from home with severe lower abdominal pain. She goes quickly to a single empty room and prepares it, collecting equipment that may be needed so that there will be no delay or unnecessary noise when the patient arrives. The night nurse realises that the symptom of lower abdominal pain without any other information could mean a variety of different conditions.

The night nurse then makes preparations for the patient to be examined and treated.

ADMISSION TO THE WARD

Pauline is brought to the ward on an ambulance stretcher and by now she is very pale and tense. John accompanies her and is obviously worried. The ambulance attendants place Pauline on the bed, and the night nurse makes sure she is as comfortable as possible before calling the duty doctor to tell him of her arrival. She then has a talk with Pauline and John, soothing their fears, and making some observations.

The doctor arrives and John is asked to sit in the waiting area with a cup of tea while his wife is examined. He is told that the doctor will see him to discuss Pauline's condition and treatment as soon as the examination is completed.

The night nurse and the doctor see Pauline together, working as a team. The doctor elicits a history from Pauline, and it becomes apparent that she has had this type of pain before, although it was right-sided the first time. She had not been to see a doctor because she was afraid that she might have to come to hospital

Physical examination reveals lower abdominal pain and rebound
Vaginal examination reveals cervical excitation and bilateral adnexal tenderness, and may reveal vaginal discharge
There is a raised white cell count and ESR

and lose valuable work time. Pauline has previously had an appendicectomy which left a large scar and which she says had 'burst' before she went to the hospital.

When the doctor has completed taking a history and doing a physical examination he diagnoses Pauline's pain as the result of acute pelvic inflammatory disease. The senior doctor on duty will be asked to confirm this diagnosis.

Cervical excitation
Fallopian tube
Ovary
Body of uterus
Broad ligament
PAIN – due to the hammer on anvil effect of the fingers pushing the cervix
Cervix
Examining fingers

The diagnosis is usually called pelvic inflammatory disease because the pelvic organs are all linked closely together and unless it is proved otherwise it is assumed that they are all inflamed. However, not all gynaecologists make this assumption so you may come across this illness called salpingitis, which means inflammation of the Fallopian tubes. For a diagram illustrating anatomical relationships in the pelvis, see p. 78.

If there is reason to suppose that the patient has an ectopic pregnancy a laparoscopy will be performed.

The duty doctor takes some blood samples from Pauline and starts giving her an intravenous infusion. When the registrar arrives he agrees that Pauline is suffering from acute pelvic inflammatory disease. There is no particular need for Pauline to undergo a laparoscopy, but in any event her previous 'burst' appendix may have left adhesions which would make this procedure hazardous.

The registrar sees John and Pauline and explains the illness and probable course of events to them. After this, John goes home and the night nurse brings Pauline a drink and helps her to settle down comfortably after she has had some analgesia. The type of analgesia given depends on the degree of pain that the patient is suffering, so that she may receive a controlled drug such as Pethidine or a much milder drug such as Paracetamol.

The night nurse carries out observations only at four-hourly intervals, to allow Pauline some time in which to rest. Pauline's full nursing assessment is postponed until morning in order to allow time for the analgesia to work and for Pauline to settle to sleep.

Initial stages

In the morning the day nurse is able to carry out a full nursing assessment in which all of Pauline's needs are noted so that a plan of care can be made. In this instance Pauline is assessed as needing pain relief which can be given in many ways including positioning the patient comfortably as well as giving the prescribed medication. She also needs help with her toilet, both because she has to rest in bed and because she is in pain and has an intravenous infusion. Pauline's appetite is poor, so one of her nursing needs is to have her appetite tempted and food presented attractively. Pauline is very anxious at the moment and needs to have all care explained to her carefully before it is given. Also she needs to be kept well informed of her progress and the likely course of events. A potential problem in Pauline's case is that as soon as she starts to feel better she may become bored; therefore the nurse will encourage John to bring in books and a tapestry kit which Pauline likes, to keep her amused.

Probable antibiotics:
The causative organism is often not found and therefore the antibiotics used are those which have effect on a wide variety of organisms. Examples of this may be Cephradine for aerobic bacteria, in combination with a drug like Metronidazole for anaerobic bacteria. These drugs are often given intravenously initially and may, variously, be given subsequently by other routes (intramuscularly, orally or rectally).

Rehabilitation

Pauline will be nursed in bed until she no longer has abdominal pain. This is a treatment based on the principle of resting any inflammatory condition, but as most people find using a bedpan difficult, Pauline will be

Sexually transmitted organisms such as *Neisseria gonorrhoeae*, *Chlamydia trachomatis*
From other lesions in the pelvis such as appendicitis, or diverticulitis
Gut organisms such as *Escheriscia coli*
From post abortal or post puerperal infections, which may have resulted from a wide range of organisms

Possible tests and medical treatment:
Blood tests – haemoglobin, full blood count and erythrocyte sedimentation rate to estimate the degree of infection. These tests will be repeated at regular intervals to monitor progress
Abdominal and vaginal examination may also be repeated to check the patient's progress
Analgesia prescribed appropriately for the degree of pain
Appropriate antibiotics
High vaginal swabs, cervical swabs and rectal

allowed up to use the lavatory. She is in no danger of pressure sores as she is able to move freely in bed, her skin is in good condition and her general health is fine. During this early phase of her treatment it is important that Pauline has her bell to hand to call a nurse if she is worried or in need of help, and that all her personal possessions are within reach.

Observations of temperature and pulse are made four-hourly, analgesia is given regularly and Pauline is observed for signs of pain in between doses of medication. There is an intravenous infusion in progress and this is checked regularly to ensure that the infusion site is not inflamed, that the infusion is running at the appropriate rate and that entries are made correctly on the fluid balance chart.

It is very important for Pauline to eat and drink while she is unwell. Firstly, this helps to combat infection. Secondly a high fibre diet and fluids will help to avoid constipation which is one of the hazards of bed rest. John is encouraged to bring any items of food or drink which might tempt her appetite to the hospital, and after the first few days Pauline is seen to be eating small but nutritious meals.

She is very anxious not to be in hospital very long so that she can get back to business. Thus one of the most important parts of her care is to help her to recognise her own health needs. Pelvic inflammatory disease can result in either an ectopic pregnancy or infertility, or the illness can become chronic, and before she leaves the hospital Pauline should not only be aware of this but have had opportunities to discuss this with John present. The continuing pain of pelvic inflammation combined with anxieties about business and the future may well make Pauline in particular need of comfort during her stay, and her nurse should ensure that she has ample opportunity to discuss her feelings. Sometimes it can be difficult

swabs may be taken to try to identify the causative organism
A midstream specimen of urine may also be collected for culture and sensitivity, to try to identify the causative organism
An intravenous infusion will be given if the patient's condition warrants it

on a busy ward to make time to sit down and talk to a patient but nevertheless this is a very important form of treatment.

The treatment starts to take effect, and as the days go by her nursing needs gradually lessen. Her pain is now evaluated as considerably improved and the analgesia is given only when needed. She is able to eat and drink, and can tolerate the antibiotics by other routes, so the intravenous infusion is discontinued. Pauline is able to walk to the lavatory and to use the bathroom without feeling pain or needing help. Thus the major nursing intervention remaining is health education. This can be started long before she goes home so that her nurse can check with her that she has understood everything.

NURSING CARE

Planning discharge

When Pauline has been receiving treatment for ten days she is sufficiently well enough to be considered for discharge home. This decision is made on the basis of her blood tests and observations which no longer show signs of infection, and of the physical examination performed by the gynaecologist being satisfactory.

Pauline and John are seen together before she is allowed home, as she must continue to rest at home, and her nurse and gynaecologist wish to be sure that she will do so. John assures everyone that Pauline's mother is coming to stay and look after her, and that he has hired some help for the business so that she will not worry about it. They are told that pelvic inflammation can recur and that it is not possible to know whether or not fertility has been affected.

Pauline takes the remainder of her course of antibiotics with her and is told that she should take Paracetamol for pain. The need for stronger pain relief would indicate that the inflammation has not completely subsided, and she should see her G.P. immediately.

Advice on discharge:

She must rest as much as she has had in hospital initially, gradually getting back to normal over the next week.

She should continue to eat and drink well.

She must remember to take the antibiotics as prescribed. It can be extremely difficult to remember to take drugs regularly once you are feeling better.

She and John are advised to refrain from intercourse until the antibiotics are completed. When sexual intercourse is resumed contraceptive measures must be taken. It should be noted that an intra-uterine contraceptive device is not considered suitable for a patient who has had a pelvic infection as this could lead to further inflammation.

Generally speaking, Pauline is reminded that her own health must not be neglected in favour of the business, and that she and John like all other human beings have a need to work, rest and experience recreation.

TEST YOURSELF

Check with your Tutor or Ward Sister that you understand the questions and have answered them fully.

1   It is said that pain is worse at night. Discuss the reasons why this may be.

2   One of the effects of inflammation is to cause an increased blood supply to the affected area. Describe the changes in menstruation that may occur.

3   What is the nurse's role in caring for a patient with chronic pain? Can you think of treatments other than analgesic medicines?

4   How may the nurse help Pauline to recognise her own health needs? What suggestions could you make to help Pauline in the future?

FURTHER READING

HACKETT, T. P. 1972. Pain and Prejudice: Why do we doubt that the patient is in pain? *Medical Times*, **99**.

JEFFCOATE, N. 1975. *Principles of Gynaecology*. Sevenoaks: Butterworths.

MCCAFFERY, M. 1983. *Nursing the Patient in Pain*. Philadelphia: Lippincott Nursing Series.

NICOL THIN, R. 1981. *Lecture Notes on Sexually Transmitted Diseases*. Oxford: Blackwell Scientific Publications.

6 Janet Black has an ectopic pregnancy

Janet and Tony Black were buying their weekly groceries on a Friday evening when Janet started to feel pain in the lower abdomen. The pain was severe enough to make her feel faint momentarily. They hurried home as soon as they could so that Janet could lie down. Once lying down, however, the pain was no better. It was a colicky pain of varying intensity, but by nine o'clock the pain was so bad that Tony took Janet to the Accident and Emergency Department of the local hospital.

Janet is 25 years old and works in an office. She and Tony have been married for 18 months and they live in a small house near the garage where Tony works as a mechanic. Janet and Tony had been using contraception up until a few months ago, but apart from attending the Family Planning Clinic, they have had very little need for medical help until now.

ADMISSION TO HOSPITAL

Once at the Accident and Emergency Department, Janet is seen and assessed by a nurse and a doctor, and routine observations made.

The doctor takes a history from Janet and makes a full physical examination. When he asks Janet about her menstrual periods she tells him that she is always irregular, and that this time her period is late as her last period was 5 or 6 weeks ago.

Observations:
Pulse
Temperature
Blood pressure
Nature and
duration of pain

The emergency doctor feels that there is a possibility that Janet has an ectopic pregnancy. He asks the duty gynaecologist to see her.

Acute and sub-acute tubal pregnancy:

Approximately 1 in 150 pregnancies are tubal and of these only 1 in 10 ruptures. However many patients are admitted with abdominal pain, and are then discovered to have a tubal pregnancy when diagnostic procedures are carried out.

Ectopic Pregnancy

Conception should take place in the Fallopian tube. The fertilised ovum is then wafted down the tube by its cilia and peristaltic action, until it is embedded in the secretory endometrium lining the uterus.

'Ectopic' means misplaced, and an ectopic pregnancy is one in which the pregnancy occurs outside the uterus. Usually, an ectopic pregnancy is sited in the Fallopian tube, as the fertilised ovum has not been passed for some reason down the Fallopian tube to the uterus. However an ectopic pregnancy may have other sites such as the broad ligament, the ovary or rarely the abdominal cavity.

Some sites of Ectopic pregnancy

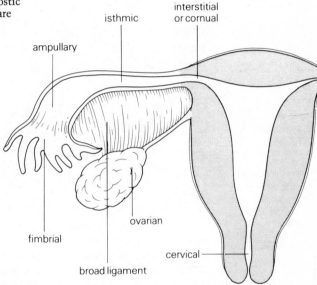

interstitial or cornual

isthmic

ampullary

fimbrial

ovarian

broad ligament

cervical

Signs and symptoms of an ectopic pregnancy:

Raised pulse rate
Low blood pressure
Temperature is within normal limits
On examination the abdomen is acutely tender
Bimanual examination demonstrates

Why is this a gynaecological emergency?

The fertilised ovum burrows into the walls of the Fallopian tube as it does into the uterus. As this happens the ovum enters its second phase of development, the trophoblast, which increases in size, and therefore there is a high risk of haemorrhage both from the invasion of the Fallopian tube walls, which contain tributaries of major blood vessels, and from the over distension of the Fallopian tube. The Fallopian tube is not the same diameter all the way down, and thus the length of time elapsing after conception and before rupture takes place

cervical excitation, with unilateral adnexal tenderness. There may or may not be a boggy swelling in one of the vaginal fornices May or may not have missed a period May have a thin dark vaginal loss, unlike menstrual flow

is variable. However it is not usually more than 6 weeks after the first day of the last menstrual period. The female reproductive organs are exceptionally well supplied with blood vessels in order to perform their normal functions.

Diagram of the Blood Supply to the Uterus, Fallopian Tubes, Ovaries and Vagina

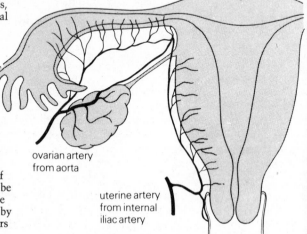

ovarian artery from aorta

uterine artery from internal iliac artery

Why does it happen?
Developmental abnormalities of the Fallopian tube Distortion of the Fallopian tubes by adjacent tumours Previous inflammation of the Fallopian tubes or to another organ in the pelvis leading to adhesions in or around the Fallopian tube. This could occlude the lumen of the tube or reduce the amount of peristaltic action of the tube The presence of an intra-uterine contraceptive device predisposes the patient to ectopic pregnancy

When the gynaecologist sees Janet he checks rapidly through the information that has already been collected and concludes by performing a bimanual vaginal examination.

Janet and Tony are seen together by the gynaecologist, and they are told that Janet may have an ectopic pregnancy and what it means. Janet will need to have a laparoscopy under a general anaesthetic to confirm the diagnosis. If the diagnosis is confirmed the gynaecologist will proceed to operate straight away. Janet and Tony are both very worried but glad that action is being taken.

Initial stages

Janet will have the minimum of preparation for the operation that is consistent with safety. Luckily she has not eaten or drunk for more than four hours so that her stomach is not full.

Janet will have her operation at 11.30 p.m. and Tony stays with her until she goes to the operating theatre. After her operation Janet will go to the Gynaecology ward, so Tony is directed there to await her arrival.

Postoperative

Janet is brought back to the ward at 12.30 a.m. by the night Sister and is received by the night nurse, who is responsible for ensuring her comfort and monitoring changes in her condition. This is done by a series of routine observations.

Once Janet has been settled into bed and made comfortable, her observations are carried out. These are all within normal limits, so, although Janet is sleepy, the night nurse allows Tony to come in and see her. In a few minutes Janet has fallen asleep and Tony goes home to bed.

The night nurse decides that her observations can be made at hourly intervals until she is sure that they are stable, and then reduced to four-hourly intervals. Janet has not needed a blood transfusion as her Fallopian tube had not ruptured. The intravenous infusion is to ensure that she remains hydrated until she is able to tolerate more than 2 litres of fluid orally over a 24 hour period. The intravenous fluid prescribed will vary according to the particular doctor's preference, but a typical prescription might be Dextrose 4.3 per cent, Saline 0.18 per cent, 500 ml in 6 hours for 24 hours, after which time the prescription will be reviewed.

Minimal theatre preparation:
Blood is taken for Hb., full blood count and cross match at least two units of blood
Identity bands are worn
Theatre gown is worn
There must be no jewellery worn except a wedding ring, which should be covered
There should be no dentures, prosthesis, or cosmetics worn
Consent form signed
Urinalysis performed
An intravenous infusion will be commenced
If there is time the upper part of the suprapubic hair will be shaved

A patient with a tubal pregnancy may have either part or all of her Fallopian tube removed. This is called respectively a partial or total salpingectomy.

**Postoperative
observations for a
patient who has
had a
salpingectomy:**
Colour
Pulse
Blood pressure
Temperature
Observing wound
site for bleeding or
swelling, this may
include
observations of
wound drains if
present
Vaginal loss
Observations
relating to the
intravenous
infusion, the rate of
the infusion, the
cannula site,
maintenance of a
fluid balance chart
Observe the
amount and timing
of micturition

Medical treatment:
Check
haemoglobin to be
sure that Janet has
not lost much
blood during or
after surgery
Listen for bowel
sounds – the bowel
has not been cut,
but it has been
handled and may
go into stasis. If the
bowel sounds are
present and Janet is
not nauseated, the
intravenous
infusion may be
discontinued
Analgesia of a
suitable strength
will be prescribed

The wound is usually a Pfannenstiel incision. This is an incision which is made transversely just above the symphysis pubis, which has the advantage of being very safe and achieves a good cosmetic result. Sometimes this incision is liable to haematoma formation, but in Janet's case the gynaecologist has decided that this is unlikely so she has no wound drains.

She has analgesia when she needs it and in the early stages of her recovery has strong medication, usually one of the controlled drugs.

Janet's night nurse has been unable to make a full nursing assessment as Janet needed to rest but during the day time her nurse is able to do so. Janet has a blanket bath and during this procedure she and her nurse are able to have a conversation where most of the information needed to formulate a plan of care is discussed. Janet is a well person apart from this operation, so her needs are centred on recovery, mentally and physically, from the effects of the operation.

Tony has brought in all of her toilet articles and night dress so she can brush her hair and clean her teeth with familiar brushes and change into her own clothes. She is helped out of bed to the lavatory and once there is able to pass urine. Her bed is made while she is up and she is glad to get back in again.

The gynaecologist arrives during the morning to discuss her operation with her, to assess postoperative progress and to prescribe any medical treatment necessary. He tells Janet that she has had one Fallopian tube removed and that she was lucky as the tube had not ruptured. She will soon recover from the operation. However, no obvious cause for the ectopic pregnancy was seen. The doctor assures Janet that it is quite possible for her to become pregnant perfectly normally after this, but that there is a slight chance that the same situation may arise. This is because the factor causing this ectopic pregnancy could lead to another.

Janet is rather distressed by this, and her nurse leaves the bed curtains drawn around her until she feels calm again. The nurse assures Janet that the doctor will be happy to talk to her and Tony together before she leaves the hospital.

<table><tr><td>NURSING CARE</td><td>

Rehabilitation

</td></tr></table>

Janet's nurse encourages her to be ambulant as much as possible and ensures that she receives enough analgesia to be comfortable while walking or sitting. Observations of temperature and pulse are made at four-hourly intervals, and the wound is checked daily. She has been told that this is a precautionary measure, to recognise any signs of infection early and give prompt treatment. A normal diet should be resumed as soon as she is able to do so, and she is encouraged to drink plenty of fluids so that her intravenous infusion can be discontinued.

<table><tr><td>NURSING CARE</td><td>

Planning discharge

</td></tr></table>

Her wound will have either silk, nylon or clip sutures, which will need to be removed before she goes home. This procedure really frightens patients who have not had sutures removed before. Her nurse realises this and tries to reduce Janet's fear by discussing the procedure in advance. In the event the sutures are no trouble at all. Recovery from this operation is rapid and Janet will be allowed out of hospital as soon as she is well and the removal of

Postoperative advice:
The wound should be kept clean
Janet should resume normal activities gradually, taking about four weeks
Sexual intercourse can be resumed when they wish
They should try to conceive again only when Janet feels mentally and physically ready to embark on a pregnancy

Signs and symptoms of a ruptured ectopic pregnancy:
Severe abdominal pain
Collapse
Rapid, thready pulse
Very low blood pressure
Skin cold and clammy
Abdomen may be distended, doughy and tender
May have air hunger

the sutures shows the wound to be well healed. The nurse and doctor talk to Janet and Tony before she is taken home five days after the operation. The purpose of this conversation is not only to give postoperative advice but also to try to bring them some comfort. Many couples blame themselves for a mishap occurring in pregnancy without there being any cause for guilt or blame, and a discussion with people whom the couple trust can sometimes reduce these feelings.

Janet and Tony leave the hospital with an Outpatient appointment to return in six weeks so that her wound can be checked and further advice given if necessary. They are determined to try for another pregnancy and the nurses who have been caring for her wish them luck as they leave.

If Tony had delayed in bringing Janet to the hospital, it is possible that her Fallopian tube might have ruptured as it does in 1 in 10 patients. When this happens bleeding can be so severe that the condition becomes fatal.

Surgery must be performed without delay, and even minimal preparations for the operation may be omitted.

However, even if the patient is moribund, once the bleeding has been arrested and the blood volume restored, recovery is rapid.

TEST YOURSELF

Check with your Tutor or Ward Sister that you understand the questions and have answered them fully.

1 Think about the way in which you would explain the condition 'ectopic pregnancy' to a patient; try it out on a colleague.

2 Janet has been described as distressed; describe her possible feelings more fully,

perhaps by discussing this with the experienced nurses on your own ward.

3   During Janet's stay she has asked when she can resume her hobby of tenpin bowling. If you were her nurse, what advice would you give?

4   The postoperative advice includes that of not having another pregnancy until they are ready. What advice do you think might also be given about contraceptive measures?

FURTHER READING

CHOO, H. O. 1974. Twin Pregnancy. *Nursing Times*, May 2nd.

FRIEDMAN, R. & GRADSTEIN, B. 1982. *Surviving Pregnancy Loss*. Boston: Little, Brown and Company.

HUDSON, C. N. 1978. *The Female Reproductive System*. Edinburgh: Churchill Livingstone.

KELLY, S. 1982. Out of Place. *Nursing Mirror*, June 30th.

7

Anne and Mike Harrison are investigated for subfertility

HISTORY

Anne and Mike Harrison did not start worrying about their childless state until Anne was 32 years old. They had both been working as teachers at the local comprehensive school until two years ago, when Anne had stopped working in order to prepare their home for a baby. The planned pregnancy did not happen.

Anne and Mike wanted to be examined and reassured that there was nothing preventing them from conceiving and bearing a child. They made an appointment with their G.P. who referred them to the Gynaecological Clinic at the local hospital.

When a couple are subfertile, both partners are investigated, although the investigation of the male partner is a simpler process than that of the female partner. The first part of the investigation is to take a careful sympathetic history and to make a full physical examination.

The male partner (History)

Details of past and any present illnesses are asked about. These may include past infectious diseases like mumps, past conditions which have necessitated surgical intervention such as hernias, undescended testes or a varicocele. Details of occupation are required as working in a hot atmosphere like a boiler house could affect the production of sperm. Social habits such as drinking alcohol can also affect the production of normal sperm. It is also important to establish that correct sexual intercourse or coitus is taking place and that the couple

Subfertility
Most healthy normal couples conceive within 12 months of trying, and a further small number of couples conceive within another 12 months. Therefore a diagnosis of subfertility is made when conception has not been achieved after 12 months of normal unprotected intercourse. Subfertility is divided into two types:
Primary means that the female partner has never become pregnant, whatever the outcome.

are trying to conceive during the female partner's most
fertile time, that is mid-cycle. The male partner must be
achieving orgasm to ensure release of semen.

The male partner (Investigation and Examination)
The doctor will be making observations all the time that
the history is being taken. He will be observing the
development of secondary sex characteristics, which will
indicate the presence of the male hormone, testosterone.
These include the normal hair distribution for an adult
male, on the face, axilla, chest, abdomen and pubis and
also the normal deep male voice.

The examination of the male partner is principally
concerned with the male genitals. They are inspected to
see if the scrotum and penis are normally developed and
for the presence of any abnormality. As mentioned earlier
these could include a varicocele, undescended testis or a
hernia.

The male partner is asked to submit a semen specimen
for testing. This may be obtained either by coitus
interruptus or by masturbation, and the sample should
reach the laboratory within 2 hours of production. Should
the couple have a moral or religious objection to this
procedure, there are other methods of obtaining the
information such as the postcoital test.

There is a wide range of normal in the tests carried out
on the sample of semen, and therefore the lower limits of
normal are those quoted. Tests are done to determine:
  Volume – which should be more than 2ml
  Sperm count – which should be more than 20,000,000
  per ml
  Motility of the sperm – which should be more than 40
  per cent four hours after production
  Normal forms of spermatozoa – which should be more
  than 60 per cent of the total
If one specimen has results which are lower than
normal, the test is repeated upon a further two
specimens, because some conditions may affect the
production of sperm temporarily.

In approximately 25 per cent of cases of subfertility the
cause is related to the male partner. In approximately 25
per cent of cases of subfertility the cause is related to the
female partner and in the remaining 50 per cent of cases
where a cause is established, it is due to a mixture of
male and female causes.

The female partner (History)
Details of past and any present illnesses are asked about.
These may include past infectious diseases such as
mumps, past conditions which have necessitated surgical
intervention such as appendicitis and the history of any
previous pregnancy. A careful analysis of the menstrual

history will be carried out, including the age at which periods started (menarche), frequency and character of menstruation, as irregular periods may indicate anovulation. Social and sexual habits will be discussed particularly with regard to alcohol intake, and frequency and timing of coitus.

The female partner (Investigation and examination)
The doctor will be making observations all the time that the history is being taken. He will be observing the development of secondary sex characteristics, which indicate the presence of the female hormones, oestrogen and progesterone. These include normal hair distribution for an adult female, absent from the face, chest and abdomen, present on the axilla and the pubic region, and also normal breast development.

The examination of the female partner includes a vaginal examination to detect any gross abnormality such as a tube–ovarian swelling. Certain tests are carried out to exclude systemic disease and these may include a mid-stream specimen of urine sent to the laboratory to exclude urinary tract infection, a full blood count to establish general well-being and a cervical smear to exclude cervical pathology. Blood tests may be taken for specific hormones to check ovulation. These are serum progesterone and prolactin, follicular stimulating hormone and luteinising hormone.

Anne and Michael are told at their initial interview that investigation of subfertility is a slow process and that they will probably be asked to attend the clinic at three-monthly intervals after the initial visits. Each step is explained to them as it happens so that they can co-operate fully in the investigation. The whole tone of the interview and all the subsequent interviews will be optimistic, not only because emotional factors are thought to have a significant role in subfertility (accounting for as many as 25 per cent of subfertility problems) but also because there are grounds for optimism. Not all childless couples can be helped to conceive but there are many who can, and about 20 per cent of all couples seeking help conceive before the tests are completed.

Anne and Michael are asked to return to the clinic in one month's time for the results of the tests which have so far been performed. In the meantime Anne is given a basal temperature chart, and asked to record her temperature as soon as she wakes in the morning. Anne is told that she should note any factor which could cause her temperature to rise such as a head cold or 'flu'.

Basal temperature chart

It is known that certain changes occur in the patient's temperature according to the hormone levels in the blood at the time. When ovulation occurs there is a slight lowering of temperature followed by a sudden rise over 24 hours. The progesterone then in the circulation keeps the body temperature up between 0.2°C and 0.5°C for the remainder of this menstrual cycle until menstruation occurs, which happens when progesterone levels have gone down.

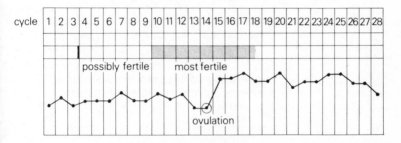

If the basal temperature chart indicates that Anne is ovulating she and Michael will be told that they need not continue to check. This is because many couples eager to have a baby become so anxious to have sexual intercourse at a time when the chart indicates fertility that a considerable strain is imposed on their marriage.

The month goes by and Anne and Michael are not sure whether to be relieved that Anne's chart looks like the example depicting ovulation, thus not needing treatment, or sorry because the cause of their problem has not been discovered. They are both glad when it is time to return to the clinic. Once there, they are told that all tests so far have been normal. The next phase of the investigation is to establish that Anne's Fallopian tubes are patent, allowing the passage of a fertilised ovum into the uterus, within the three days needed for it to become embedded.

There are two tests commonly used to establish tubal patency one of which can be performed as an outpatient investigation.

Hysterosalpingogram

A hysterosalpingogram is an X-ray taken after radio-opaque media has passed through the uterus and Fallopian tubes. This demonstrates the shape of the uterine cavity and the shape, direction and patency of the Fallopian tubes. Unfortunately, this may be painful, is very expensive and is not completely reliable. This test does not reveal the presence of endometriosis which is associated with subfertility nor can the ovaries be examined. Sometimes the radio-opaque media acts as an irritant to the Fallopian tubes causing spasm and giving an appearance of tubal blockage which is incorrect.

This test is not therefore as popular as it was before the advent of laparoscopy and dye insufflation.

Laparoscopy and dye insufflation is a procedure in which approximately three litres of carbon dioxide are pumped into the peritoneal cavity of the anaesthetised patient so that the anterior abdominal wall is lifted away from the organs of reproduction and a clear view obtained. Two small incisions are made, one usually low down in the abdomen for the passage of the gas and the other usually through the lower rim of the umbilicus to pass the laparoscope. This is a small slim fibre optic telescope which gives a good view of the pelvic organs. A dye solution is passed through the Fallopian tubes and its exit can be observed through the laparoscope. Any hindrance to the passage of the dye can be seen, as can any pelvic sepsis, endometriosis, and the ovaries. The incision through which the laparoscope has passed is usually sutured with one suture which can be removed 1–5 days later. The patient may have abdominal pain after this procedure and may also have shoulder pain from the collection of any unexpelled gas under the diaphragm giving referred pain. This gas becomes absorbed in a matter of days.

Another test of ovulation may be performed at the same time as a laparoscopy, a dilatation and curettage. This is performed to compare the state of the endometrium with the date of the patient's last menstrual cycle, giving information about her ovulation and hormone levels.

A post-coital test is one in which the female patient has her cervical mucus examined between 6 and 24 hours after coitus has taken place. This is done to see that the spermatozoa are motile and invading the cervical mucus, as they should be. Many remedies are offered if there is said to be cervical hostility, among them hormone treatment to render the cervical mucus thinner and more easily penetrated.

Anne's gynaecologist explains the test to her in detail and makes an appointment for her to be admitted to the Gynaecological ward on a date in the latter half of her menstrual cycle. The state of her endometrium should then be glandular and dense demonstrating the presence of progesterone.

Meanwhile there is another test that can be done to see whether or not her cervical mucus is hostile to Michael's sperm, as can happen. This test is called the post-coital test.

Their post-coital test is explained to them carefully. The test proves normal and they are both now becoming apprehensive lest there is no remedy for their childless state.

Anne is admitted to the Gynaecological ward on a busy day when there are several other patients being admitted.

ADMISSION TO THE WARD

Observations:
Temperature
Pulse
Blood pressure
Date of last
menstrual period

The first three of these observations are taken to provide a baseline for comparison with the observations which will be made after the operation. The date of the last menstrual period provides a check that Anne has

A nurse introducing herself as Liz Parker shows Anne to a bed and explains the nurse call system to her. Anne is given plenty of time to unpack and to change into her night clothes. This is the usual procedure to be followed even though Anne is not ill, because there will be various examinations prior to the operation and these will be easier if Anne is wearing clothes which can be taken off easily. Liz makes some observations explaining the reasons for them as she does so.

Liz makes a full nursing assessment by discussing Anne's needs with her. Anne is a well woman and her main requirements are preparation for the operation and information. She has had most of her queries answered by the gynaecologist in the clinic but coming into hospital has made her so nervous that she feels the need for further reassurance. Liz gives her all the information that she is able to and makes a note on the care plan that she is come to the hospital at the right time of her cycle particularly nervous so that Sister and the doctor can continue to reassure her.

NURSING CARE

Initial stages

Anne is introduced to the other patients in her room and they all have a cup of tea together. The atmosphere in the ward becomes quite cheerful, but the nurses working here know that there are many ways for a patient to demonstrate nervousness and are alert for signs of stress. Stress may be demonstrated in many ways, withdrawal, tearfulness and aggression among them. Should any of these be observed the nurses will offer comfort and support, and if unsuccessful they have a range of people to ask for additional help depending on the nature of the problem causing the stress.

Later that day other preparations for the forthcoming visit to the operating theatre are made. Anne has a specimen of urine tested, she is seen by the gynaecologist and the anaesthetist and feels a little more relaxed by the time Michael comes to visit her in the evening. When it is time to settle down for the night Anne is offered a mild sedative in order that she may have a good night's rest as many patients find it difficult to sleep in hospital, especially before an operation.

The next morning the last preparations for theatre are made. Anne is feeling pleasantly sleepy from her premedication when she is escorted to the theatre for a laparoscopy and dye insufflation with a dilatation and curettage.

This reveals that both of Anne's Fallopian tubes are surrounded by adhesions and that there has been no spill of dye from the fimbrial ends of the tubes.

Rehabilitation

Anne returns to the ward via the recovery area, and is pleased to see a nurse she knows accompanying her back to bed. Unfortunately Anne vomits a small amount of fluid as soon as she is moved into bed. She is offered an anti-emetic injection which she accepts, and it soon stops the nausea. There are several different anti-emetic drugs which could be prescribed and patients tend to vary in their response to them.

Liz makes several postoperative observations while the injection takes effect, hoping that if all is well Anne may rest undisturbed until the nausea has gone.

Observations:
Pulse
Blood pressure
Vaginal loss
Observation of both wounds, that is the wound by the umbilicus and the stab wound through which the pneumoperitoneum was achieved.

Anne's observations show no sign of haemorrhage, which is the main danger. She is left undisturbed with a clean vomit bowl in case she feels sick again, and her nurse call bell within easy reach.

When she wakes her first thought is for the result of this diagnostic procedure. Her second, however, is that she has quite severe pain both in the abdomen and in her left shoulder, so she calles a nurse. Anne is given an analgesic, in this case Paracetamol with a drink as she no longer feels sick. Stronger analgesia may be given but Paracetamol is usually effective and does not make the patient sleepy. Anne is told that if she remembers to breathe in and out deeply and to move about as much as she can the gas will disperse and the pain will go.

When the analgesia has had time to work Anne is helped to have a wash, clean her teeth, and brush her hair. Her morale is raised by putting her own nightdress back on and by being allowed out of bed for the first time. Liz walks with her to the lavatory so that help can be given if she shows signs of weakness, and after passing urine, she is helped back to bed. At the moment she is not told of the operation findings because it is thought better that the gynaecologist who performed the test and her nurse will tell her together so that the possible forms of treatment available to her can be fully discussed. Most patients need telling more than once and the anaesthetic itself is partly to blame for this, in making patients forgetful. However the staff accept that this is a necessity and repeat the information as often as it is needed.

Tubal surgery varies according to the nature of the malfunction. A patient who has had a sterilisation with clips has a simpler operation with a better chance of success than a patient who has had tubal sepsis. Patients who have had tubal surgery have a high rate of ectopic pregnancies and only about 1 in 4 of those who have had previous pelvic sepsis will conceive at all.

Planning discharge

Michael comes to visit her in the evening and the doctor and nurse see them together to discuss the future. They are told that Anne could have her Fallopian tubes operated on to try to restore function.

They are also told that she is very unlikely to conceive unless surgery is performed. Two options remain: one is to adopt a child and the other is for a doctor in a specialised centre to attempt in vitro fertilisation. Anne and Michael have heard of test tube babies but know very little, never having thought it might apply to them (see concluding chapter). The gynaecologist tells Anne and Michael all he can to help them to make a decision regarding their future, and gives them time to decide. After he has gone Liz sits with them for a while answering further questions. Michael is reluctant for Anne to undergo further surgery especially with such a slim chance of success, while Anne feels that any chance of having a baby of their own naturally is worth a try.

Anne continues to need analgesia until the next day but says that the pain is gradually improving. She has come to a decision and finally sleeps well. When the doctor comes to the ward to see if Anne is well enough to go home she tells him that she and Michael have decided that she should have tubal surgery. An appointment for readmission is made for her and she is allowed to go home as both the doctor and the nurse are satisfied that she is well after the operation. Liz makes sure that Anne understands the advice given to her when she is ready to leave the hospital.

Advice on discharge:

She should not undertake any strenuous physical activity for at least a week

She should attend her G.P. surgery for removal of the suture in a few days' time

She should use sanitary towels rather than tampons for her next period

Her next period could be either early or late

She should continue to use analgesia until she no longer needs it, in accordance with the instructions on the bottle, although it is expected that she will no longer need anything after a few days

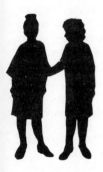

Michael comes to collect Anne and they both say farewell to her nurses, making jokes about 'the next time'.

The relationship that Anne has with the nurses is important because she is returning for much more extensive surgery the next time. It will be of real benefit to her if she is able to come back to a familiar welcoming environment with people that she knows and trusts.

The wait to come back to the hospital can be a very trying time for some women, as they are usually eager to 'get it over with'. Sometimes the ward nurses can help by suggesting ways of keeping the patient's mind off the subject, such as going away on a visit if the circumstances are favourable, or they may help by simply giving as much information as they possibly can.

Check with your Tutor or Ward Sister that you understand the questions and have answered them fully.

1   What effects may continuing infertility have on a couple? Discuss this with the qualified nurses on your own ward.

2   Anne has been told that her G.P. will remove her stitch. What effect could this have on other patients in the community? Can community services in your area cope with the demands imposed on them by patients having early discharge from hospital?

3   How would you explain to Anne the reason for her shoulder pain?

4   Infertility is often thought by the lay public to be a woman's problem only. Discuss both sexes' reaction to being told that they need to be investigated for infertility.

FURTHER
READING

COWPER, A. 1982. Time and a Word. *Nursing Mirror Clinical Forum*, April 14th.
INTERNATIONAL PLANNED PARENTHOOD FEDERATION. 1979. *Handbook of Infertility*. IPPF.
JEFFCOATE, N. 1975. *Principles of Gynaecology*. Sevenoaks: Butterworths.
REYNOLD, M. 1984. *Gynaecological Nursing*. Oxford: Blackwell Scientific Publications.

8 Mary Day has a hysterectomy

Mary is 40 years old and has two sons aged 18 and 20 years respectively. She has been divorced for two years and she and her sons live in a house near the park.

The trouble started a few months ago when her menstrual periods became markedly heavier and contained clots. Initially she thought that this would cease naturally and must be related to the menopause. However the heaviness of the flow was getting worse month by month to the point that Mary had to spend some part of her period lying down, usually the 2nd and 4th days.

When Mary attended the clinic for the first time the gynaecologist asked her many questions about her general health, her social history and the history of her menstruation. A vaginal examination was also performed. and the gynaecologist discussed his findings with her. She was told that her uterus was enlarged and though it seemed likely that this was due to fibroids, it would be advisable for her to come into hospital and have a dilatation and curettage in order to confirm the diagnosis. Mary is not too surprised, she has several friends who have mentioned having fibroids to her and the term is familiar to most women who read women's magazines. Mary is not absolutely sure of the correct meaning so the gynaecologist explains it to her.

Fibroids are more properly called fibromyoma. They are benign new growths arising from the muscle wall of the uterus. The troublesome symptoms that they cause are related almost entirely to their position in the uterine wall and it is from this that they are classified. Fibroids

Treatment for fibroids: Fibroids regress after the menopause so that if the symptoms are not severe, the fibroid is not large and the patient is near the time of the menopause, it may be best to leave the fibroid untreated. If the patient is pre-menopausal and wants to have children, the gynaecologist may offer a myomectomy, which means removal of the fibroid leaving the uterus. However, fibroids can recur and as a general rule the uterus should not be operated upon too often in a patient who wishes to become pregnant as it weakens the uterine wall. If the patient is postmenopausal or has completed her family she will probably be offered a hysterectomy.

Conditions which may cause menorrhagia:
Dysfunctional uterine bleeding
Adenomyoma
Pelvic infection
Presence of an intra-uterine contraceptive device

very rarely become malignant. The symptoms caused by fibroids are complex and those below are a guide:

Types of fibroids

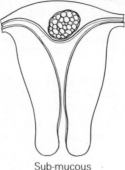

Sub-mucous

An increased area of endometrium leads to symptoms of menorrhagia. Sub-mucous fibroids account for only 10 per cent of the total.

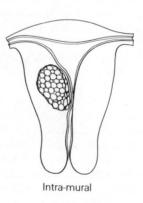

Intra-mural

There is an increase in surface area of endometrium which may lead to menorrhagia. Intra-mural fibroids account for about 70 per cent of all fibroids.

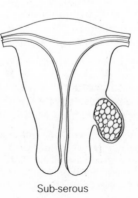

Sub-serous

Sub-serous fibroids give rise to a variety of symptoms. It must be remembered that fibroids may occur in large numbers and at a variety of sites all at the same time. Also, fibroids may be 'pedunculated' i.e. on a stalk.

Carcinoma of the
cervix or
endometrium
Blood dyscrasias

The gynaecologist explains to her that there are other conditions which may cause similar symptoms and he tells her what these are.

Mary now has a dilatation and curettage which confirms the presence of several fibroids and she has accepted the plan of hysterectomy.

ADMISSION TO THE WARD

Once Mary has been fully admitted and introduced to the other patients she feels quite at home because she has been a patient on this ward recently and is familiar with the staff and all the ward routine. Liz Parker has discussed with her in detail not only the pre-operative preparation for this operation but also the postoperative care. Most importantly she has made sure that Mary's ideas about the operation are correct ones. This is one of the operations where the patient may suffer by having a great deal of misinformation as there are many myths about hysterectomy. Sometimes patients get their information from relations who had their operations many years ago when the anaesthetic and operative conditions were less sophisticated than they are today. In order to give accurate information the nurse must know which type of hysterectomy is to be performed.

Types of hysterectomy:
Sub-total hysterectomy – Removal of the body of the uterus leaving the cervix
Total hysterectomy – Removal of the entire uterus
Total hysterectomy and bilateral salpingo-oophorectomy – Removal of the entire uterus, both Fallopian tubes and ovaries
Wertheim's hysterectomy – Removal of the entire uterus, both Fallopian tubes and ovaries, the upper one-third of the vagina, the pelvic lymph nodes and paracervical tissue
Vaginal hysterectomy – Removal of the entire uterus via the vagina
In the premenopausal patient the ovaries are only removed if absolutely necessary as their removal leads to a premature menopause.

Pre-operative preparation for a patient undergoing a hysterectomy:

Full information must be given

The patient may be seen by a physiotherapist to be instructed in exercises for the postoperative period

Blood will be taken to check the patient's fitness for the operation by a full blood count, and blood will be cross matched so that there will be blood available if the patient has an excessive blood loss during or after the operation.

Preparation of the patient's bowel will vary according to the surgeon's wishes, some believing that no preparation should be made if the patient has had her bowels opened in the past 24 hours, while others think that various types of enemata are appropriate. If the bowel is full, the surgeon may accidentally perforate it due to its proximity to the operation area

Preparation of the patient's skin, which includes a thorough shave and a bath pre-operatively

The patient's urine is tested for abnormalities

The patient has baseline observations made

The patient is weighed, as it may be relevant to the dosage of drugs prescribed

---

NURSING CARE

Initial stages

During Mary's full nursing assessment Liz has already asked her about her home, family and activities, so that the best after-hospital care can be planned. For instance it is important to know if Mary has large numbers of stairs to climb, or if she has small children or animals to look after when she gets home. It is also essential to know about Mary's leisure activities so that suitable advice can be given. Many women in her age group are far more active than they would have been only a generation ago, and in different ways such as attending aerobics classes. Mary says that both her sons help her with the household chores. She has thought about the time when the operation is over and she will leave the hospital again, and says that if at all possible she would like to go to a convalescent home for a while. Patients having a hysterectomy are often in hospital only a short time, 6–8 days, so that plans for their discharge from hospital start as soon as they come in. The nurse may need to educate the patient and her family about the activities of daily living and how to recognise complications should they occur. Specific detailed instruction must be given, and it should be given more than once, preferably supplemented with some written material for the patient to refer to.

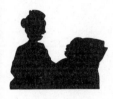

Mary is having her operation in the afternoon, so she has a light breakfast of tea and toast at eight o'clock and then tries to snuggle down and go back to sleep. It is a very long morning although when they can the nurses try to stop for a chat. When her nurse tells her to bathe and dress in a theatre gown, it is a great relief.

An hour before the operation Liz comes and askes her to pass urine so that she will be comfortable in bed while the premedication takes effect. When she has done so, Liz, who is accompanied by a staff nurse, returns with her premedication. In this case the anaesthetist has prescribed Papaveretum and Scopolamine intramuscularly. The staff nurse explains that the syringe has two substances in it and that one of them will make her mouth very dry and the other will make her rather sleepy. Once the injection has been given, Mary is made comfortable, with her call bell close at hand. She is asked not to get out of bed as her legs may feel weak after the injection, but to call instead.

It seems to Mary a very short space of time before the theatre porters and Liz are taking her to the theatre. Here Liz gives her hand a squeeze and says a cheery 'see you later' to Mary as she hands over Mary's care to the nurse in the anaesthetic room. Today Liz as part of her ward learning programme has the opportunity to watch the operation so she goes quickly to the changing room to change into theatre clothes. An understanding of gynaecological nursing is greatly enhanced by observation in the operating theatre and the Outpatient Department.

NURSING CARE

Rehabilitation

Mary awakens while Liz and the theatre porters are taking her back to the ward. As soon as Liz notices that she is awake, she tells Mary that the operation is over and that they are taking her back to bed. Once there Liz helps Mary into a comfortable position carrying out routine observations as she does so. She looks at her colour and ensures that the wound site is not bleeding and that the amount of vaginal loss draining onto the sanitary towel is not excessive. There is no specific posthysterectomy position, but the patient will be comfortable and safe in the event of vomiting if she is lying in the lateral position with her knees slightly flexed and her head resting on one pillow. Sometimes it helps the patient to have a pillow supporting her abdomen or one placed behind her back. Once Mary has settled down Liz carries out the remaining observations of pulse, blood pressure and respirations, which are within normal limits. They are then taken half-hourly until they have been stable for at least two hours after her return to the ward. Mary does not require an analgesic or an anti-emetic, but Liz checks the chart to see that they have been prescribed so that there need be no delay when Mary is ready for some.

Postoperative nursing in major gynaecological surgery is largely prophylactic. This operation has been carried out in an extremely vascular area so that one of the complications to be watched for is that of haemorrhage. Two of the organs closely linked to the uterus and the vagina are the bowel and the bladder, and although they have not been cut, they will have been handled and will react accordingly. The bowel may exhibit a degree of stasis so that there is a risk of paralytic ileus. The bladder may exhibit a degree of stasis so that there is a risk of retention of urine.

The patient has had a disruption to the pelvic blood supply so she is in some danger of deep vein thrombosis. All patients having surgical procedures have a certain amount of pain and it is known that hysterectomy patients complain of pain in the wound site initially, and suffer from pain in the abdomen generally in the succeeding days that is described as 'wind' pain. Again all patients having an operation may succumb to an infection and because of this it is usual for prophylactic antibiotics to be given. It should be remembered that patients who have had a hysterectomy have two wounds leading to the surface, one in the lower abdomen and the other at the vault of the vagina and that both need care. Some women also experience mood swings after this operation although other women are so relieved to be rid of the cause of long-standing problems that they experience no mood swings at all. The nurse should be sensitive to the patient's moods and feel able to discuss them with her if she desires this. Women of other ethnic groups, notably African women, view hysterectomy as the end of their lives as women and may become very distressed.

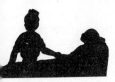

Mary's care plan recognises the points mentioned above. Her observations are gradually reduced to four-hourly, and each time the dressing is inspected for drainage. Mary has no wound drains to be checked. During the first morning after surgery she is given a blanket bath and a vulval washdown; she also has help with brushing her hair and cleaning her teeth.

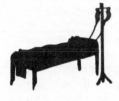

She has not been nauseated so she is allowed to have a cup of tea. When her oral intake approaches 150–180 ml of fluid hourly when awake and her bowel sounds are assessed as normal, the intravenous infusion will be discontinued.

Mary sits out of bed while her bed is made, and then her nurse takes her for a walk as far as the lavatory. Once there Mary finds that although she would like to pass urine she cannot. Liz tries leaving her on her own with the water turned on gently, and then tries running warm water over the vulva, but to no avail. Liz tells her that it often takes time for the bladder to work properly after the operation and that all will be well by later that morning. When she is back in bed, Mary complains of some abdominal pain. Having noted that Mary had received analgesia three hours ago, Liz decides to report this to Sister. It seems possible that Mary has a full bladder as she has absorbed fluid from the intravenous infusion and orally. Another possibility is that Mary has suffered some damage to the ureters at the time of surgery as the ureters run one each side of the cervix and can be difficult to dissect free. If this was the case Mary would be producing urine but it would be escaping into the peritoneal cavity.

Sister and the doctor are coming round to see all the patients who have had surgery on the preceding day anyway so Liz tells Mary that they are coming and that her pain will be resolved soon. The doctor explains to Mary that the operation went well and that she had a huge fibroid; he also examines her. This includes listening to bowel sounds in case she has a paralytic ileus and percussing the bladder to detect whether or not she has a full bladder. Bowel sounds are listened for through a stethoscope, but percussion is carried out by listening to the resonance or dullness heard when the doctor taps the fingers of one hand with the other while moving the hand across the abdomen. Dullness indicates that there is fluid beneath. Mary has a full bladder and the doctor congratulates Liz for making the inference that the pain was due to this rather than a lack of pain relief. The doctor suggests that a urinary catheter be passed to drain the bladder. Away from Mary's bedside Sister asks Liz if she has passed a urethral catheter before, and on being told that she has not, arranges that a staff nurse should demonstrate this to her. Mary is rather apprehensive about this procedure but it is explained in detail before it is started. Afterwards she is much more comfortable and is able to have a nap. Liz asks the physiotherapist, who is seeing all the patients, to leave Mary until last so that she can rest before doing exercises.

By the evening of her first postoperative day the intravenous infusion is removed and she has been up to the lavatory and successfully passed urine. She still needs help to get out of bed and to walk but Liz can see that she is making excellent progress. Mary has also eaten a small meal; Sister prefers patients to have a small solid meal than a very liquid meal like soup and jelly as she believes that this helps to avoid the 'wind' pain.

Mary has her haemoglobin checked to see that she has not lost much blood during or after surgery, and this proves to be similar to her pre-operative haemoglobin. Mary is gradually ambulated throughout the rest of her hospital stay. During this postoperative period she has a vaginal loss that is bright red to start with and then turns brown. Mary is shown how to use the bidet so that she feels happy about her cleanliness and also so that there is less risk of any discharge becoming infected. She is also encouraged to have a bath with assistance once the first 24 hours after surgery are over. Most patients are nervous about this and prefer to wait longer but there are no grounds for believing that baths are harmful as the wound is sealed after 24 hours. Mary has clips to the wound which are removed after four days to ensure a good cosmetic result.

Planning discharge

The only time that Mary feels depressed after this operation is when she sees that the other patients have all got their husbands or boyfriends visiting, as she has not really yet become accustomed to the idea that she is divorced. However when her sons arrive they make her laugh painfully with tales of their cooking disasters and they manage to come every evening. Unfortunately this does make her worry about them when they have left for home and she is left with little to think about. One evening after the visitors have gone home Liz notices that she is lying quietly in bed instead of joining the usual ward chat, so Liz sits with her for a while. Mary soon confesses that she is worried her sons will do something really disastrous while she is away at the convalescent home. Liz lets her talk about it and later tells Sister. Sister knows that it would be quite easy for Mary to talk herself out of going away to convalesce as she feels well in hospital with very little to do, and a speedy return to all her normal chores would be very bad for her.

Sister is very experienced in getting patients to discuss their problems and is soon able to elicit from Mary that she is not only worried about the boys coping without her but is homesick and afraid that she will have no visitors and be lonely at the convalescent home. Sister persuades Mary to go if her younger sister, with whom the boys get on well, will call in at home several days a week. Sister also makes a note to tell Mary's sons that Mary will still need to be visited while she is away.

When the time comes for Mary to leave the hospital for the convalescent home she has a momentary panic about meeting all the new staff, but the nurses manage to reassure her. She is well enough to have a change of scene as she is now getting bored with being in hospital.

Mary has been given a lot of advice about her recovery from the hysterectomy and is feeling confident about what to expect.

Advice given on discharge:

She will feel very tired initially and should try to rest with her feet up in the afternoons for the first few weeks. It is expected that she will no longer need to do this after about four weeks

She should let her body be the guide in knowing how much activity to take; walking is good, but she should try to walk where there would be somewhere to sit should she feel tired

She should not drive a vehicle for about four weeks as the footwork required can be very tiring for her abdominal muscles

Her vaginal loss should tail off within a couple of weeks and if it does not or it becomes bright red again or smelly, she should seek help from her G.P.

She should not have sexual intercourse for at least four weeks after the operation

There is no reason for her to gain weight unless she eats too much without taking sufficient exercise. Only if her ovaries had been removed would she expect to have menopausal symptoms such as hot flushes.

Liz accompanies her to the hospital transport to say goodbye and Mary says she will come and see them all when she returns to the clinic for her postoperative appointment in six weeks' time.

Check with your Tutor or Ward Sister that you understand the questions and have answered them fully.

1 Sister and the doctor were very pleased that Liz had correctly interpreted the cause of Mary's pain as being due to a full bladder. Describe the course of events if this had not been diagnosed.

2 What old wives' tales are there about hysterectomy? Discuss ways in which we can educate the patient about these myths.

3 Discuss Mary's possible emotions as opposed to those described.

4 If Mary had decided to go straight home following this operation what Social Services/family resources might have been mobilised to help her?

FURTHER READING

JEFFCOATE, N. 1975. *Principles of Gynaecology*. Sevenoaks: Butterworths.

LLEWELLYN-JONES, D. 1978. *Fundamentals of Gynaecology*. London: Faber and Faber.

ROBINSON, J. 1983. Like a Foreign Country. *Nursing Mirror*, July 13th.

WEBB, C. & WILSON-BARNETT, J. 1983. Hysterectomy: Dispelling the Myths. *Nursing Times Occasional Papers* 1 and 2, **79** (30).

9 Ellen Taylor has a prolapse

Ellen Taylor is 68 years old and lives with her two cats in a bungalow. She has three grown-up daughters and one grown-up son and numerous grandchildren, and they come to take her out for the day quite often.

Lately however, Ellen had not been as keen on outings as she used to be, and it took her daughters some time to find out why. The truth was that Ellen was suffering from stress incontinence of urine, which meant that any exertion like coughing or laughing would cause her to lose some urine. Thus she was always preoccupied with carrying sufficient clean underwear to change and about becoming smelly. Even at the bungalow her much loved gardening had become a chore and a source of worry because of this problem.

Ellen's daughter accompanies her to their G.P. who makes an appointment for her to attend the Gynaecological Clinic. Once there Ellen is asked questions about her general health, social history, menstrual history and about the history of the stress incontinence. A vaginal examination is performed and the gynaecologist tells Ellen that she has a prolapse. He says that it is possible for this condition to be treated medically with a ring pessary which when inserted vaginally will hold the prolapse up and will stop the incontinence. However these have to be changed every six months and it is usually thought better for the patient if surgery is performed, providing that the patient is well otherwise. Ellen is quite

Predisposing factors in vaginal prolapse:
This is more common in the post menopausal age group as there is less oestrogen in circulation and the tissues become less elastic
Having many babies or large babies stretches the supports of the uterus and vagina
Any condition which causes an increased intra abdominal pressure such as chronic cough, chronic constipation or an abdominal mass
Consistently lifting heavy weights

keen to have the operation as she does not like the idea of the six-monthly change of pessary and is not worried by the thought of the operation. She is given an appointment to be admitted to the hospital for an anterior vaginal repair or vaginal colporrhaphy. The gynaecologist explains this to Ellen in as much detail as he can.

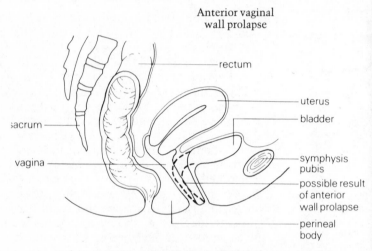

Anterior vaginal
wall prolapse

rectum

uterus

bladder

sacrum

vagina

symphysis
pubis

possible result
of anterior
wall prolapse

perineal
body

This diagram shows a projected bulge forward of the anterior vaginal wall. This is usually separated into prolapse of the upper vaginal wall which takes with it the closely associated wall of the bladder and is called cystocele, and prolapse of the lower part of the vaginal wall taking with it the urethra, which is called a urethrocele.

Most patients complaining of a prolapse say that they have a feeling of a lump coming down. They also often have backache. Urinary symptoms such as stress incontinence can occur due to weakening and displacement of the sphincter mechanism of the bladder.

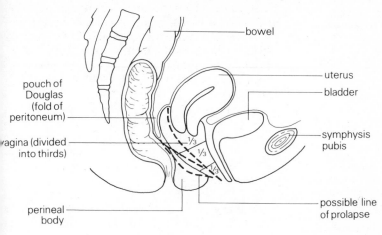

Posterior vaginal wall prolapse

- bowel
- uterus
- bladder
- symphysis pubis
- possible line of prolapse

pouch of Douglas (fold of peritoneum)

vagina (divided into thirds)

perineal body

$^1/_3$ $^1/_3$ $^1/_3$

This diagram shows a projected bulge forward of the posterior vaginal wall. This is usually separated into: prolapse of the upper one-third of the vagina which takes the small bowel into the Pouch of Douglas, and is called enterocele; prolapse of the middle third of the vagina which takes with it the associated structure of the rectum and is called rectocele; and lastly prolapse of the lower third of the vaginal wall. This last part of the vagina is guarded by the perineal body so that prolapse here can only occur if there is a deficiency of the perineum due to trauma or childbirth. Posterior wall prolapses cause few symptoms unless they are sufficiently large to cause bowel problems.

ADMISSION TO THE WARD

Ellen is brought to the hospital by one of her daughters, who stays to get Ellen settled in, helping her to unpack. She also answers some of the questions asked by Liz Parker, who introduces herself as her nurse. Liz anticipates that Ellen will need more help from the nursing staff than younger patients, and collects

Procidentia:
Prolapse of the uterus is always accompanied by prolapse of the upper vagina. Three degrees of uterine prolapse are recognised:
The first degree is when there is slight prolapse of the uterus but the cervix is not visible at the vaginal orifice.
The second degree is when the cervix is visible at or beyond the vulva but reduces spontaneously.
The third degree is when the body of the uterus lies outside the vagina altogether and does not reduce spontaneously, this is also called a complete procidentia.
The symptoms caused by a procidentia vary according to the degree of prolapse, from backache to the oedema and infection resulting from complete procidentia.

quite a lot of information with which to formulate a plan of care. Ellen is shown round the ward and introduced to some of the other patients, most of whom are young and who obviously feel that they ought to look after Ellen.

Liz discusses with Ellen and her daughter the pre-operative care and the likely course of events postoperatively so that Ellen will not be nervous about anything and will be able to cooperate in her own care. However Ellen does not seem particularly interested and Liz, although puzzled by this, ascribes it to nervousness.

Liz has also discussed with her, during the nursing assessment while her daughter was still there, Ellen's home circumstances, her family and her hobbies with a view to deciding what after hospital care would be the most suitable. It seems that she will be well cared for at her daughter's home for some time after the operation. The usual hospital stay after a vaginal repair is about 7 to 14 days. During this time Ellen will receive specific detailed information about her recovery, and as she will be staying with her daughter, her daughter will be included in the discussions. Information is also given about the action to take in the event of any complications.

Pre-operative preparation for a patient undergoing a colporrhaphy:

Full information must be given, to promote patient cooperation and reduce anxiety

The patient should be seen by a physiotherapist who will be helping her to exercise in the postoperative period

Blood will be taken to check that the patient is fit for the operation by doing a full blood count, and usually blood will be sent to the laboratory so that serum will be held in case an urgent cross match becomes necessary

Preparation of the patient's bowel will be carried out and this varies from doctor to doctor. Some will request that the patient receive an enema and some suggest a mild aperient only in the day before the operation

Preparation of the patient's skin, which includes a

thorough shave and a bath pre-operatively
Urine is tested pre-operatively for abnormalities
Baseline observations are made
The patient is weighed, so that the correct dosage of
drugs can be calculated

NURSING CARE

In anterior colporrhaphy the anterior vaginal wall is incised and redundant tissue excised. At the same time the vesico–vaginal fascia is exposed and is then picked up on both sides by stitches which will bring the fascia together to make a support for the bladder and the urethra. The incision is then repaired.

Buttressing of the bladder neck is done to relieve the symptom of stress incontinence. Three or four sutures are inserted into the pubo-cervical fascia specifically at the level of the bladder neck (urethro-vesicular junction) to elevate, support and tighten the bladder sphincter.

Initial stages

Ellen is quiet for the rest of the day, but her nurse thinks this is because it takes a while to settle down. She is very distressed when she comes on duty the next morning and hears from the night nurse at the report that Ellen has been 'difficult', apparently ignoring what is said to her and being 'in the way' when the night nurses were busy. Ellen's operation will take place later that morning and she is allowed nothing to eat or drink for at least six hours beforehand. Thus Liz is surprised to see her take a boiled sweet from her locker, and stops her just in time from eating it. During the conversation that follows it soon becomes apparent that Ellen cannot hear properly and is lip reading a lot of the time, a fact which was masked by her daughter's presence yesterday. She does not have a hearing aid and is not aware of how little she can hear. Liz spends some time with Ellen carefully going over the information that was given yesterday and the vital information for today, double checking that Ellen understands before reporting to Sister. Sister is extremely pleased that this discovery has been made as she says that patients are rarely 'difficult', there is usually a reason why they behave in a manner which seems inappropriate. She records the information on the nursing assessment so that other nurses coming on duty will be aware of Ellen's hearing disability and then makes a note to discuss with the doctor a referral to the ear, nose and throat consultant when Ellen is well enough after this coming operation.

Eventually the time comes for Ellen to have the last preparations made for theatre; she has a bath, puts on a clean gown, and passes urine before being given a mild premedication. An hour later she is wheeled down to the theatre for an anterior colporrhaphy and buttressing of the bladder neck.

<table>
<tr><td>

NURSING CARE

</td></tr>
</table>

Rehabilitation

Ellen is returned to the ward and made comfortable in bed. There is no specific postoperative position but like other gynaecological patients it is better not to elevate the foot of the bed unless it is vital to increase the blood supply to the brain. This is because blood may collect in the vagina and give a misleading impression of the amount of blood loss a patient is having. Liz takes routine postoperative observations, and uses the opportunity to see whether there is vaginal loss. The readings are all close to Ellen's baseline observations so their frequency will be gradually reduced until they are made every four hours at which time her temperature will also be taken. As the upper vagina has a relatively poor nerve supply an anterior colporrhaphy is not unduly painful, but Liz checks her prescription chart to ensure that Ellen would be able to have an analgesic or an anti-emetic should she require one.

There are many similarities between the postoperative care of a patient who has had an anterior colporrhaphy and a patient who has had a hysterectomy.

As this is a very vascular area, some gynaecologists insert a vaginal pack to help maintain haemostasis, which will remain in place for 24–28 hours. The uterus is more closely associated with the bladder than with the bowel and therefore Ellen has a catheter draining her urine continuously. Retention of urine would otherwise be likely to occur due to local oedema and the tightening of the bladder sphincter. The catheter will remain in 2–5 days depending on the gynaecologist's preference. Some gynaecologists use a supra-pubic catheter for this purpose both because there is less danger of an ascending urinary tract infection and because it facilitates checking for restoration of bladder function. Patients with a urethral catheter who need to have a residual urine estimate have the catheter removed, pass or attempt to pass urine, and then have the catheter re-inserted, thus allowing the possibility of ascending infection to occur. Patients with a supra-pubic catheter who need to have a residual urine estimate have the catheter clamped, pass or attempt to pass urine and then have the catheter unclamped. The residual urine is that which is left after the patient has passed urine.

The bowel is not likely to go into stasis and therefore as soon as Ellen feels able to eat and drink she will be encouraged to drink about 150–180 ml of fluid hourly when she is awake. This will ensure that she does not become dehydrated as she has no intravenous infusion. 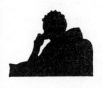 It is also important that Ellen drinks well so that there is a good flow of urine through the bladder helping to avoid urinary tract infection, and a high fluid intake also helps to avoid constipation. Ellen will be encouraged to choose and eat high fibre items from the menu so that the risk of her straining at stool and putting pressure on the suture line is minimised. Her intake and output are recorded so that a balance can be maintained.

Some doctors consider an intravenous infusion necessary in order to restore fluid volume rapidly in case of haemorrhage, or to keep the patient well supplied with fluid during the initial post-anaesthetic period.

Ellen is at risk of a deep vein thrombosis and needs to be mobilised as early as possible.

Her observations will eventually be reduced to twice daily if all is well. The presence of a vaginal pack and catheter were explained to her pre-operatively and again today, but like many patients she finds these hard to accept. It bothers her that she does not need to go to the lavatory to pass urine and she is frightened of wetting the bed. Liz remembers to stand facing the light so that Ellen can lip read and repeats the information to her until it seems that she understands.

Ellen is very thirsty by the morning after the operation and has a cup of tea and breakfast cereal with milk to start the day, so it seems unlikely that she will have any difficulty in drinking enough.

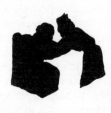

She is given a blanket bath and is encouraged to wash her face and arms herself. It is vitally important that patients are not allowed to become dependent on assistance, especially older patients who will return to living alone after leaving the hospital. Ellen sits out of bed to clean her teeth and brush her hair, and goes for a walk around the ward. When the doctor comes to see her, however, she is back in bed, having become rather tired. The doctor examines her to see that she is recovering from the operation and the anaesthetic, and explains what has taken place. Liz listens carefully to this as she knows that Ellen will not comprehend all the information at once and that she is the person in the best position to repeat it and ensure that Ellen understands.

At the end of the first postoperative day Ellen has been out of bed several times, she has drunk a good volume of fluids and begun to eat well. Her daughters have been to visit and are delighted with her progress. They have brought her lots of tit-bits to eat, magazines and Get Well cards made for her by her grandchildren, who were not allowed to come today. Many hospitals permit open visiting but the nurse should always be guided by the patient's condition in allowing visitors. In Ellen's case Sister knows by long experience that by the end of the first day she will be very tired, and perhaps her grandchildren had best not visit until a few days' time.

<table>
<tr><td>NURSING
CARE</td></tr>
</table>

Planning discharge

Ellen continues to make good progress and once she has had the vaginal pack removed 24 hours after the operation, she is allowed to bathe with help. No antiseptic lotion or other preparation has been added to the bath water, just some bath foam that she has been given, and Ellen thoroughly enjoys it. Later she is shown how to use the bidet. Removing the vaginal pack is not a difficult procedure but it should be performed as an aseptic technique and the patient should be rested in bed afterwards, with her vaginal loss checked frequently. When a vaginal pack has been removed there is a possibility that the removal will disrupt the suture line or reveal a bleeding point, and frequent observation ensures that prompt action can be taken if this is so. The catheter is cared for by cleaning around the urethral orifice and using aseptic technique when changing the catheter bag. Many gynaecologists request that the catheter be clamped and released at set intervals prior to removal to improve bladder tone; others do not consider this to be of value. Ellen's catheter is removed on the fifth day after the operation, early in the morning, which allows plenty of time during the day to establish normal micturition. She succeeds easily on her first attempt to pass urine although as she only passes 100 ml at once Liz suspects that she may not have completely emptied her bladder. Each time she passes urine it is measured, and in the evening of that day a residual urine estimate is carried out. This proves to be 50 ml, which is considered to be good, and her urinary output is no longer measured.

Ellen has had her haemoglobin checked since the operation and it is close to her pre-operative level. Each day she is visited by the physiotherapist who encourages her to do some gentle pelvic floor exercises to minimise the risk of a recurrence of the prolapse.

She continues to make good progress and is ready to leave hospital by the seventh day after the operation. She has been well prepared for her discharge home, as has her daughter. Before she leaves the hospital the gynaecologist performs a vaginal examination to be sure that no adhesions have formed in the vagina, that there is no haematoma, and that healing is taking place.

The physiotherapist has said goodbye. Ellen has an appointment to see the ENT Consultant to investigate her deafness and an appointment to return to the Gynaecology Clinic in six weeks' time, so it only remains to ensure that she has understood the advice she has been given and to say goodbye.

Advice on discharge:

She will feel tired and should rest with her feet up each afternoon, gradually increasing the amount of time she is active until by the fourth week after leaving the hospital she no longer needs afternoon rests.

She does not drive so the fact that she is advised not to drive for four weeks is no problem to her.

She may expect no more than a small amount of brownish or pinkish vaginal loss which should gradually diminish.

Sometimes patients see a remnant of a suture on their pad when they are changing. This is not anything to be alarmed about as it is the superficial part of the suture coming away once the suture starts to dissolve.

Symptoms of a urinary tract infection can be discussed so

that should one occur it may be treated without delay. She must not strain her pelvic floor muscles and this means that she must not lift anything heavy (which for this purpose may be defined as that which takes two hands to lift). She must avoid straining at stool and should have any cough treated.

Ellen will have the wound examined after six weeks when she returns to the clinic and if all is well she need no longer take these precautions.

If Ellen had been having sexual intercourse prior to the operation she would have been advised to refrain until told at the clinic that she could resume.

<table>
<tr><td>

TEST YOURSELF

</td><td>

Check with your Tutor or Ward Sister that you understand the questions and have answered them fully.

1 Try to think of other ways in which a patient's senses might have become impaired, and which might escape detection until the patient is among strangers?

2 Can you think of any possible risks in Ellen going to stay with her daughter who has been described as slightly dominating? What are they?

3 How would you explain this operation with its attendant pack and catheter to a patient?

4 Some patients do not like to bathe as often as daily. As we think that bathing is an essential part of the wound care after vaginal repair, what action would you take to encourage them to bathe?

</td></tr>
</table>

FURTHER READING

BALFOUR, P. B. 1979. Operative Management of Vaginal Prolapse. *Nursing Times*, June 7th.
LLEWELLYN-JONES, D. 1978. *Fundamentals of Gynaecology*. London: Faber and Faber.

Cathy Reed has an abnormal cervical smear

Cathy Reed is 26 years old and she and her husband Martin have 3 children of 8, 6 and 4 years old. They live in a small house with very few amenities. Martin's job does not earn him enough to consider buying their own house so they are awaiting rehousing by the council.

Cathy had attended the Family Planning Clinic as a routine visit and while she was there a cervical smear was taken. Cathy was not worried by this as she had had one taken before and regarded them as routine. She did begin to worry a week later when her G.P.'s receptionist telephoned to ask her to come to the surgery to discuss the smear result.

Cervical cytology: Cervical cells can be examined by collecting the cells as a cervical smear. With the patient in the dorsal or lithotomy position, a speculum is passed in order to visualise the cervix. A spatula is rotated around the external os of the cervix and exfoliated cells are collected and smeared onto a slide to be sent to the laboratory.

The purpose of cervical cytology screening is to detect premalignant conditions of the cervix (i.e. abnormal change that is limited to the surface epithelium only, which, untreated, would lead to invasive cancer of the cervix).

By detection and treatment of such affected women it is hoped that the incidence of carcinoma of the cervix itself can be diminished. At present the DHSS only recommends routine cervical screening on women aged 35 years or over and for such smears to be repeated no more frequently than 5 yearly. However it is now apparent that the age incidence of premalignant change and of carcinoma of the cervix is falling, and that the

Colposcopy is used to assess the site, size and extent of the lesion diagnosed by the cervical smear. Representative biopsies are then taken and further treatment planned (see also concluding chapter).

change from premalignant to invasive change can occur more rapidly than in a 5 year span. Many therefore feel that current DHSS policy needs modification.

Her G.P. tries to allay her fears by telling her that the cervical smear showed some slightly misshapen cells (dysplasia) and he thinks that she should be seen by a gynaecologist in order to determine whether or not she needs further tests or treatment. An appointment is made for her at the Gynaecology Clinic where she has a colposcopy. Subsequent to this, an appointment is made for Cathy to be admitted to the hospital for a cone biopsy.

Cone biopsy of the cervix

A cone biopsy is one where a cone shaped piece of tissue is removed from the cervix to take out previously identified abnormal cells. The procedure is a simple one but is carried out under a general anaesthetic and requires the patient to be observed for a period after the operation. In most instances it is thought preferable for the patient to remain in hospital for 24–48 hours. The main hazard is that of haemorrhage from this very vascular tissue.

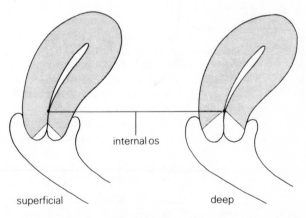

internal os

superficial   deep

Cathy is told that she can expect to come into the hospital on the day before the operation and to remain in the hospital until at least the day after the operation. She agrees to this because she has a sister-in-law who will take

Carcinoma of the cervix is classified by its invasion and spread from the cervix. In 95 per cent of cases the diagnosis is squamous cell carcinoma and in the remaining 5 per cent it is adenocarcinoma. Invasive cancer of the cervix is treated by a combination of radiotherapy and surgery.

care of the children for her. It would be very difficult for Martin to take time away from work to be at home during the week. The gynaecologist and the clinic nurse have answered all of her questions during the clinic visit, and a full physical examination and history have been taken. Many illnesses have factors in common which are known to predispose to them, and this is so of carcinoma of the cervix.

Factors predisposing towards cervical carcinoma:
Early age of first coitus
Multiple sexual partners
Multiparity
Being in a low socio-economic group
Viral as in the link between squamous cell carcinoma and Herpes type 2 virus and viral warts
Male factors – certain semen may lead to abnormal change in dividing cervical cells.

Cathy's condition is premalignant and the cone biopsy will be carried out to ensure that no abnormal tissue remains to become malignant.

ADMISSION TO THE WARD

Cathy makes all her arrangements for coming into hospital and then waits for the day to come. She is not particularly worried about the admission as all three children were born in hospital. She is very worried, however, about the result of the operation.

On the day of her admission, Cathy arrives at the ward and is shown to her bed by Liz Parker. She is then asked to change into her nightclothes and shown where to unpack her belongings. This is a busy day on the ward and she is placed in a room where women are recovering from operations the day before. She finds this reassuring as the patients seem cheerful and the nurses look confident and unhurried. Shortly Liz comes back and Cathy's baseline observations are made. They discuss her needs while in the hospital so that her nursing care can be planned. Cathy is physically well apart from the result of the cervical smear so her needs are primarily those related to her operation. She is also worried about the children so as Liz shows her around the ward she points out where Cathy can telephone home for news. Liz also explains the ward routine to her and assures her that the children will be allowed to visit. Cathy was advised to stop taking the contraceptive pill when she attended the clinic as taking it pre-operatively can put the patient at risk of deep vein thrombosis.

Liz discusses with her in detail all the pre-operative care she will be given and what to expect postoperatively. In this way Cathy will fear the unknown less and will be able to cooperate in her care.

NURSING CARE

Initial stages

Cathy gradually becomes familiar with the ward, the nurses and the other patients. She is seen by the gynaecologist and the anaesthetist to ensure that she is well enough for the operation and the anaesthetic. At visiting time Martin brings the children to see her, and she feels cheered by this even though they are not encouraged to stay long for fear of disturbing the postoperative patients in the same room. That night Cathy accepts a mild sedative to ensure a good night's sleep, and she is surprised at how well she slept when morning comes. As the operation is an early one, she is not allowed anything to eat or drink, and is soon made ready for the operating theatre.

An hour later she is taken to the anaesthetic room. She is unaware of events until she is being helped back to bed after the operation. Liz tells her that she is back in bed and makes her comfortable, checking the sanitary pad for blood as she does so. Routine postoperative observations are carried out at half-hourly intervals initially and will be reduced to four hourly when her condition is assessed as being safe by the experienced ward nurses.

Liz also checks the prescription chart in case the doctor has prescribed any medications and to ensure that an analgesic and anti-emetic are prescribed in case of need. This operation is not usually painful but the patient may have a headache or other mild pain that an analgesic could alleviate.

Should a patient experience a haemorrhage in the postoperative period, two modes of treatment are available. If the bleeding is moderate to heavy a vaginal pack is inserted, which will act as a pressure dressing. Correctly inserted vaginal packs exert sufficient pressure on the vaginal wall to make it very difficult for the patient to pass urine, so a urinary catheter will be used. The pack and the catheter will be removed after 24–28 hours and the patient observed on bed rest for some hours after their removal. If the bleeding is severe the patient may be taken back to the operating theatre so that bleeding points can be sutured under a general anaesthetic.

| NURSING CARE |

Rehabilitation

Cathy's condition is assessed as being sufficiently stable to reduce the frequency of her observations to four-hourly. In the evening her husband visits, but she is still very sleepy and apart from delivering Get Well cards that the children have made and giving her their love he does not talk much. It is enough to be able to hold hands and to know that all is well so far.

In the morning Cathy feels wide awake and eats a full breakfast before being escorted to the lavatory to pass urine. She has been advised that she may experience some blood loss in the lavatory which will probably be due to blood pooling in the vagina while she was lying down rather than being fresh blood. Her nurse stays well within calling distance though, just in case all is not well. Cathy feels rather weak and tired by the time she has done this and had a wash in the bathroom, so she is glad to get back to bed for a while. The doctor calls to see her to be sure that she is recovering from the operation and the anaesthetic. He is not able to assure her that the operation is a total success until the laboratory has processed the tissue, but he is able to tell her that he is confident all the abnormal cells have been removed on the basis of the colposcopy findings.

Planning discharge

The doctor tells Cathy that she may rest as much as she likes today and that she may be allowed to go home on the following day. All the results should be available in about a week's time, so before she goes home she will be given an appointment to return to the Outpatients Department then.

Cathy enjoys the remainder of the day, being able to rest away from the children, and by evening is feeling considerably better. Sister realises that she will have difficulty in resting at home with three young children and suggests that Cathy's sister-in-law might be asked to continue helping with the children for another week.

The following day Cathy is able to leave the hospital. The nurse and the doctor see her before she is allowed home to ensure that she is well enough to go and also that she has understood the advice that she has been given.

Advice on discharge:

Dark brown or pinkish vaginal loss may be experienced for a few days and is normal. However, should the character of the vaginal loss change to become either bright red or offensive-smelling, she should seek advice quickly

She should not use internal sanitary protection until after her next menstrual period

She should refrain from sexual intercourse for at least a month as the danger of secondary haemorrhage is greatest between 10 and 14 days after the operation. She is also reminded that extra contraceptive precautions are necessary until she has recommenced taking the contraceptive pill for at least one cycle

She should not do any strenuous activity for about a month

TEST YOURSELF

Check with your Tutor or Ward Sister that you understand the questions and have answered them fully.

1 Consider and describe ways in which to break bad news to a patient.

2 What nursing action should be taken if Cathy has a heavy vaginal blood loss postoperatively?

3 Postoperative infection may lead to secondary haemorrhage, what nursing intervention would help to prevent this?

FURTHER READING

BRITISH SOCIETY FOR CLINICAL CYTOLOGY. 1981. *Taking Uterine Cervical Smears.* Aberdeen: University of Aberdeen Press.

GARREY, M. W. *et al.* 1978. *Gynaecology Illustrated.* Edinburgh: Churchill Livingstone.

TINDALL, V., YULE, R. & HUNTER, R. 1984. Cervical Cancer (series of 5 parts). *Nursing Mirror*, started Oct. 3rd.

Alice Stewart has a vulval carcinoma

Causes of vulval swelling:
An injury leading to haematoma formation
An infection such as a labial abscess
Enlargement of Bartholin's gland such as a cyst
A benign neoplasm
A cyst such as sebaceous or retention cysts
Malignant neoplasm

Signs and symptoms of vulval carcinoma:
Pruritus vulvae – itchiness of the vulva
Soreness or pain usually in a specific area
Changes in colour
The appearance of a lump
Bleeding or offensive discharge from the lump

Alice Stewart is a well 78 year old who lives with her husband George in a rest home, pleasantly situated outside the town. George is an ex-carpenter, a spry active 79 year old. They have no children as their only son was killed in the Second World War.

She has been experiencing some joint stiffness lately and Mrs Gable, the owner of the rest home, has had to help Alice to climb in and out of the bath. On one occasion she notices that Alice has a red swelling on the vulva. Mrs Gable tells her that she thinks the doctor ought to see the lump and rather reluctantly Alice agrees.

Mrs Gable takes her to the G.P.'s surgery in the car and once there the doctor tells Alice that he cannot be sure what exactly has caused the lump and that she needs to be seen by a gynaecologist. An appointment is made for a few weeks' time.

While waiting to attend the hospital, Alice and George discuss the possibilities and they both feel that the lump must be cancer. This makes Alice very reluctant to attend the hospital as she feels that she will be persuaded into having an operation that she does not want. The reason for her reluctance is that she has had several friends who have needed surgery and who have never really recovered their full strength. George however does not share her views and says that his life would not be worth living without his Alice and that she must attend and do whatever the doctor tells her to do, so that she can be well.

It is usual to take
**biopsies from
several sites**
because vulval
carcinoma can be
multi focal

She agrees to go, and on the morning of her appointment Mrs Gable drives them both to the hospital. The gynaecologist takes a full history and examines Alice physically, and when he has done so he tells Alice that she needs to come into the hospital and have a biopsy of the lump performed. Alice, knowing what George will say, agrees to this and is given an appointment to be admitted in two weeks' time. At that time, she is admitted to the hospital and has several vulval biopsies taken. She returns home to await the outcome of the tests.

ADMISSION TO THE WARD

The result of the biopsies is squamous cell carcinoma of the vulva and this is explained to her, and a radical vulvectomy arranged. Alice is admitted to the ward several days before her scheduled operation so that she can be prepared mentally and physically for it. Mrs Gable drives Alice and George to the ward where they are met by a nurse. Alice is escorted to her bed and the nurse asks her to unpack and change into her nightdress. George stays with her while the nurse takes routine baseline observations. The nurse notes Alice's joint stiffness during the nursing assessment and makes a special mention of it on the care plan. George is impressed by the nurse's warmth and understanding, and in due course he and Alice are given a cup of tea. Eventually George and Mrs Gable have to go home, and Alice is introduced to the other patients. She remembers her way around the ward from her previous visit for the biopsies.

Her nurse and the gynaecologist visit to discuss with her the operation and the pre-operative care. Alice also must see the physiotherapist and have some tests, both of which will happen on the following day.

Initial stages

Alice finds it difficult to sleep that night; she has refused a sedative and finds the ward noisy and the bed strange. It is also the first time she has been separated from George for many years. The next day she is very tired and as soon as possible, Sister moves her into a single room, so that she can rest.

This is a mutilating operation which will alter Alice's appearance in the vulval area considerably once the wound has healed. There is no way to make the shock of this easier to bear except by considerate preparation and winning the patient's trust so that she can confide her feelings in us. The nearest equivalent operation is mastectomy after which patients worry not only about carcinoma but about their appearance as a woman. Mastectomy however has become a problem widely talked of in the popular press and for which self-help groups have been formed, while patients having vulvectomy bear this alone or with a partner. Each patient reacts in an individual manner and some will need more help than others.

On the morning of the operation Alice is awakened early and assisted to bathe by Liz who has noted that her joint stiffness makes bathing difficult. Alice puts on a clean theatre gown and receives her premedication. She relaxes and lies quietly until Liz and the theatre porters take her to the anaesthetic room where she is anaesthetised.

Radical vulvectomy

A wide local excision is made because although slow
growing the tumour spreads to become locally invasive.
Lymph nodes in the groin area are excised because the
tumour spreads to local lymph glands

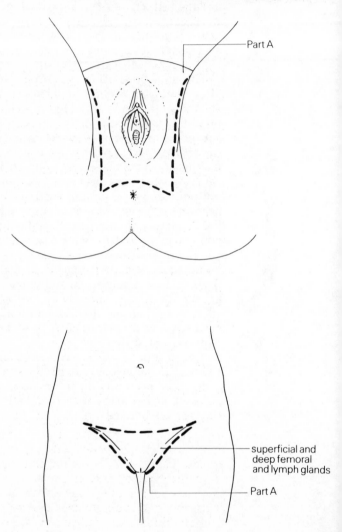

Part A

superficial and
deep femoral
and lymph glands

Part A

Rehabilitation

Alice returns to the ward and is made comfortable in bed. There is no specific postoperative position following vulvectomy but this operation has been carried out in an area which is particularly difficult to keep pressure free, so great care is needed. Once she has been made comfortable, her nurse takes routine observations and inspects the wound dressing for oozing. Alice's preliminary observations are satisfactory and her nurse decides to continue taking them half-hourly until they are stable and have returned near her baseline observations. Although this operation is extensive it is not as painful as one might expect; nevertheless her nurse checks the prescription chart to see if any treatment has been ordered and to ensure that an analgesic and an anti-emetic have been prescribed should Alice need them. It is usual for prophylactic antibiotics to be given, intravenously in the first instance.

Alice has returned from the operation with drains to the wound site. These are usually Redivac drains to remove the fluid which drains copiously from this type of wound for a considerable time. The fluid is serosanguinous at first and later will become serous only. These are vacuum drains and it is important that the suction is maintained, although this is sometimes difficult as they lie quite near the surface.

She also has an indwelling urinary catheter which prevents her from suffering retention of urine or risking urine being spilt on the wound. This is usually on free drainage.

An intravenous infusion is in progress as there is a considerable loss of fluid during the operation, and she may need a blood transfusion. Her fluid balance must be monitored on a chart which is kept accurately. Alice is unlikely to have her bowels open until several days after the operation, and thus may need a stool softener such as Milpar.

She is an elderly lady and will need to be ambulated early to prevent several complications. This is very difficult to do, because of the wound drains and the presence of the intravenous infusion, but it is essential. A patient having a vulvectomy is at considerable risk of deep vein thrombosis and pressure sores and the best method of avoiding these complications is frequent movement.

Care of the wound can present some problems as there is profuse drainage. The wound should have a non-adhesive dressing left intact as long as possible, and one way of coping with the fluid exuding from the wound is to use pads which allow outward passage of fluid only, held in place with elasticated pants. Once the initial period is over Alice will be encouraged to bathe with assistance and will have her dressing reapplied after the bath. It is important that the bath be cleaned before and after she uses it.

The physiotherapist will supplement the early mobilisation with exercises, and in order to achieve the maximum amount of movement as well as the maximum amount of comfort, a carefully judged dose of analgesia will be given.

Alice's observations are soon reduced to four-hourly observations. The presence of the vacuum drains, catheter and intravenous infusion were explained to her preoperatively and again after the operation. She is encouraged to drink and has a cup of tea on the morning after the operation without feeling nauseated.

The doctor comes to see her on the morning after the operation and tells her that all has gone well. There was a large amount of drainage overnight and the Redivac bottles are changed; the dressing, however, is clean and intact. Alice is receiving antibiotic drugs through the infusion tubing, which is inspected frequently to ensure that the cannula site is not inflamed and that the infusion is running according to the time prescribed. She is given an analgesic, so that she is not afraid to move and is then helped to have a full blanket bath. In order to maximise her independence she is encouraged to do as much for herself as possible, including cleaning her teeth and brushing her hair. Alice copes with all the tubing fairly well and is able to go for a short walk later in the day with a lot of assistance. Such mobilisation helps to give her a change of position, encouraging her to breathe deeply and avoiding slowing down of the circulation in the lower limbs. She feels proud of herself for having walked on her first postoperative day and seems well on her way to recovery.

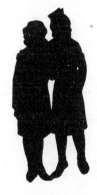

Alice is reluctant to drink very much on her first postoperative day and it is several days before she is ready to eat a meal.

Information given to her in the first few days after the operation will need to be repeated at intervals as she will probably not absorb it all initially. She is very tired after her first day and although George comes to sit with her for a while she is too exhausted to talk. George feels happier just to see her even with all the tubing, which can be very disturbing to the observer.

Throughout the rest of her stay Alice makes slow but steady progress. This is an operation which takes a long time to heal partly because it is extensive, partly because it is difficult to keep sterile, and partly because the wound edges may become devascularised. It is the rule rather than the exception that some or all of the wound breaks down, needing to have the dead tissue removed before healing can take place. The wound care and assessment are a crucial part of the nursing given to Alice.

The intravenous infusion is removed after

several days when Alice is able to drink sufficient fluids to make a balance with the fluids
she is losing. Once the intravenous infusion is
completed the prescribed antibiotic drugs
have to be given by other routes. She is gradually mobilised so that four days after the
operation she is ambulant with help to get in
and out of bed. She now starts having baths
twice daily with the dressings being renewed
after each one. The vacuum drains are removed one by one as soon as the drainage
lessens. Her catheter remains for two weeks
and is cared for meticulously so that the risk of
ascending infection is reduced.

Alice begins to manage regular bowel action
each day and the timing of her baths takes this
into account. However she needs a good deal of
help and encouragement to choose and eat a
nourishing and high fibre diet. George is always trying to think of ways to tempt her
appetite which is capricious. He is sometimes
successful and sometimes not. She is becoming increasingly bored with being in hospital.

Until the wound requires only two dressings a
day, however, she needs hospital care, as community nurses have difficulty in providing a
more frequent service than this. All the staff
try to think of things which will keep her
interested, and ask for help from the occupa-
tional therapist, but in fact Alice prefers activities which she can see are useful to the nurses,
like stamping menu cards with the name of
the ward.

Her nurse has tried to recognise the moment
when Alice would be ready to see the wound,
and obviously this is better done when the
wound is nearly healed. In the event Alice
takes it quite well and asks if her dressings can
be removed when George next comes so that
he can be shown too. She is concerned for his
reaction, 'because men are such babies'. Her
nurse agrees to this and removes the dressing

before visiting time, waiting ready to replace it when they have finished looking. Alice and George are both a little emotional after this, but by the following day they say it could have been worse, and have apparently accepted it.

NURSING CARE

Planning discharge

When the day comes that Sister tells Alice that her wound is well enough healed for arrangements to be made for discharge home, Alice is overjoyed. It is arranged that the community nurse should call and dress the wound twice a day and that Alice should have an outpatient appointment for two weeks' time.

Alice has been in the hospital for six weeks, which is a long time for her to be away from her home and a long time for a patient to be on a Gynaecological ward. All the staff have become very fond of Alice, she has been so gallant and cheerful during this difficult time.

Before Alice leaves the hospital, she and George are given a lot of advice. Because Mrs Gable looks after the couple to a certain extent, at their wish she is included in their discussions. Finally all that can be said has been said, and Mrs Gable takes Alice, George and a mountain of books, cards and possessions home.

The prognosis for Alice is quite good. The five-year survival rate is 50–60 per cent of all cases treated and is as great as 70–80 per cent in cases where the lymph nodes are not involved.

Advice on discharge:
She will feel very tired and should rest with her feet up for some time each afternoon. She should try to be active during the other parts of the day.
She should continue to eat a balanced diet, and to clean herself gently but thoroughly after each time she uses the lavatory.

The community nurse will call every day to observe the wound and assess progress and to report to the doctor. She is not taking any medication.

She and George should not attempt sexual intercourse until the wound has fully healed. It should be noted that this information may or not be important to the couple, and this should be elicited before such advice is given.

<table>
<tr><td>

TEST YOURSELF

</td><td>

Check with your Tutor or Ward Sister that you understand the questions and have answered them fully.

</td></tr>
</table>

1   Describe Alice's reactions to the sight of the wound as they might have been rather than as they were described here, and any nursing action you can think of that might help to reduce the shock to her.

2   Alice is slightly older than the average age for a gynaecology patient. What difference does this make to her nursing care?

3   There are many ways of promoting wound healing. Describe those that may be useful for a patient with a radical vulvectomy.

4   Alice will be well cared for when she goes home. What Social Services might be able to help the patient who is less well cared for?

FURTHER READING

BAILEY, R. & GRAYSHON, J. 1983. *Obstetric and Gynaecological Nursing* (Nurses Aids Series). Eastbourne: Baillière Tindall.

GOODMAN, M. 1984. Caring for Laser Vulvectomy Patients. *Nursing Mirror Clinical Forum*, **159** (3).

JEFFCOATE, N. 1975. *Principles of Gynaecology*. Sevenoaks: Butterworths.

12 Conclusion

Gynaecological nursing is constantly changing both in the technical achievements which now help us to care for our patients and in the way our patients are changing as a response to a changing environment. Women today are coming to expect equality and are becoming better informed about their bodies and the health services available to them.

Gynaecological nursing has become recognised as a specialist nursing topic. There is now an English National Board Approved Course in Gynaecological Nursing for those qualified nurses wishing to extend their knowledge and skills. There is also a forum for gynaecological nurses within the framework of the Association of Nursing Practice.

Three of the technical advances which are changing the nature of gynaecological nursing today are the use of the colposcope, the laser and the development of in vitro fertilisation.

The colposcope is an optical instrument used to examine the patient's cervix. It is a low-powered binocular instrument which is used in conjunction with the technique of cervical cytology. Colposcopy can be performed by skilled gynaecologists in the Outpatient Department and can be used with the laser to eradicate abnormal cells identified on cervical smear.

Laser stands for Light Amplification by Stimulated Emission of Radiation. The carbon dioxide laser vaporises tissue so that tissue such as cervical intraepithelial neoplasia can be removed painlessly and completely under the enhanced vision of the colposcope. The fact that the procedure is painless means that women can be treated as outpatients which is easier and more convenient for them. Most forms of treatment to the cervix involve some risk of haemorrhage, but the laser has a sealing effect on the blood vessels and the risk of bleeding is thus greatly reduced.

In vitro fertilisation is a development to help infertile couples to have children. There are at present few centres which offer this service.

In vitro fertilisation, sometimes called by the media test tube babies, is a method by which women, who are ovulating but unable to conceive due to tubal blockage, may be helped to conceive outside the body. The patient is given a drug to ensure that she has more than one ova ready for fertilisation (usually Clomiphene). The ova are collected by needle aspiration under scan control or under direct vision with the laparoscope. The male partner's semen, after preparation, is added to the ova, and the container is kept at body temperature while fertilisation takes place. The fertilised ovum begins to mature and at a certain stage of cell division is placed inside the uterus where it is hoped that the fertilised ovum will embed.

There have been many successes using this technique both in the United Kingdom and elsewhere, notably the United States of America and in Australia.

This technique, while giving hope to many women formerly considered infertile, has also brought with it a number of ethical dilemmas. For example, should extra embryos be grown for research purposes? Should a woman be able to bear another woman's child? What are the rights of the embryo?

The Warnock Committee has reported and made recommendations to the Government in 1984 and legislation is expected.

There are also many new and enhanced treatments in use for patients with malignancy. Cytotoxic therapy and radiotherapy have considerably improved both in efficacy and in diminishing of their side effects but it is beyond the scope of this book to discuss this in detail. However most wards now would be involved in the preparation of a patient for transfer to a ward which specialises in oncology. Patients should be given as much information as possible on the likely course of events and helped to accept the treatment. One condition which has been mentioned in this book which would necessitate the patient having a radium implant is cervical intraepithelial neoplasia which is invasive cancer of the cervix.

The first part of treatment for a patient who has been diagnosed to have this condition is to establish exactly how far the tumour has spread. This is divided into categories 1, 2, 3 and 4 with Stage 1 being that where only the cervix itself is affected through to Stage 4 where there has been metastatic spread.

If a patient is to be told that she has a neoplastic disease it may be helpful to have her husband or close friend with her. Certainly this diagnosis should be relayed by someone who is sympathetic to the patient and will leave her time to accept the news. Once the information has been assimilated the future course of events can be explained and the patient allowed all the time she needs to ask questions.

Giving information to a patient who has carcinoma is always a very sensitive issue, as some patients do not wish to be told and some wish to know but do not wish for their families to be told. Many patients sense that they have a malignant growth but do not want to hear it put into words. It may be that nurses, who after all are the members of the team spending the largest amount of time with the patient, are the best people to know to which category a particular patient belongs.

Much has been said about nursing and social change, but not as much, perhaps, about the ways in which gynaecological nursing expects to be involved in this.

One of the changes which is taking place this decade is the introduction of Well Woman Clinics. These were specifically designed to cater for women in groups considered to be at risk, such as those in lower income brackets. The sort of service that is being offered is screening and prevention, for example breast checks, cervical smears, etc. and to this end much health education is being devoted.

Research has indicated that a very high proportion of women attending a Well Woman Clinic are worried about aspects of their health that come under the heading of gynaecology although it would be fair to add that there are other topics of worry such as weight problems.

Research has not indicated, however, that the type of patient the clinics were designed for actually attends. The person attending is far more likely to be someone who is already well aware of the services available and of health education.

Self-help groups are also another relatively new form of therapy. These are usually associations of people who have as their common bond similar types of distressing experience so that the members give each other mutual support. There may or may not be a health care professional as part of the group, but in any event the help being given is not medical. It is more the discussion and advice that any upset person can get from another who has suffered in the same way. In the gynaecological field there are now self-help groups for patients who have had a miscarriage and those who have had a hysterectomy. Addresses for the local branches of these should be available on your gynaecology ward.

Many of the social changes that are affecting gynaecology are related to women's perceptions of menstrual disorders and childbirth. As you may know pregnancy is considered to be a gynaecological condition if there is a problem before the 28th week of pregnancy and an obstetric condition thereafter.

Research has indicated that many women perceive doctors as treating pregnancy as a medical problem rather than as a joyful natural occasion taking place in the context of the woman's life. Women want more information about what is happening to them as well as more control over their care. In gynaecological nursing only those pregnancies causing a problem are seen; however it would be foolish to imagine that for this reason we can ignore the feelings and wishes of so many women. Many have their menstrual problems described as psychosomatic or psychogenic, and the quality of treatment is variable. It is difficult to relate these feelings to a patient's care on the Gynaecology ward as any patient admitted to hospital for a menstrual disorder is obviously being taken seriously. However medical literature is full of examples where doctors experience difficulties in the treatment of menstrual disorders and premenstrual syndrome, and have made some very unfortunate statements. Women today will no longer tolerate this, and all efforts should be made to help patients to have the care that they want and need.

Great attempts are being made in nursing to ensure that all patients are as well informed as it is possible for them to be and are not spoken to in a way that belittles them. All patients should be nursed as individuals with a past, present and future, and one tool that helps us to view the patient in the context of their lives is the nursing process.

Patients are no longer seen by their medical problems, such as 'the hysterectomy in the corner bed', but as individuals, with a full recognition that they have status, family responsibilities and a life apart from their current health problem.

A constant awareness of the changes in technology and society are necessary, in order for nursing to change in response. Good nursing care can only come through the efforts of individual nurses to relate theory to practice.

FURTHER READING

BARRETT, M. & ROBERTS, H. 1978. *Women, Sexuality and Social Control.* London: Routledge and Kegan Paul.

HUNTER, R. 1984. Cervical Cancer Treatment Techniques. *Nursing Mirror,* **159** (14).

LENNANE, J. 1982. *The Changing Experience of Women.* Milton Keynes: The Open University.

OAKLEY, A. & GRAHAM, H. 1982. *Women, Health and Reproduction.* London: Routledge and Kegan Paul.

REYNOLDS, M. 1984. *Gynaecological Nursing.* Oxford: Blackwell Scientific Publications.

WINSTON, R. 1984. Test Tube babies. *Nursing Times,* July 18th.

INDEX